HORIZONS IN WORLD CARDIOVASCULAR RESEARCH

HORIZONS IN WORLD CARDIOVASCULAR RESEARCH

VOLUME 17

Horizons in World Cardiovascular Research

Additional books and e-books in this series can be found on Nova's website under the Series tab.

HORIZONS IN WORLD CARDIOVASCULAR RESEARCH

HORIZONS IN WORLD CARDIOVASCULAR RESEARCH

VOLUME 17

ELEANOR H. BENNINGTON
EDITOR

nova
Medicine & Health
New York

NOTICE TO THE READER

Library of Congress Cataloging-in-Publication Data

ISBN: 978-1-53616-157-1
ISSN: 2157-6130

Published by Nova Science Publishers, Inc. † New York

CONTENTS

PREFACE

Atrial fibrillation is initiated by triggers in combination with underlying atrial substrate. Horizons in World Cardiovascular Research Volume 17 discusses how innovations in cardiac magnetic resonance imaging techniques, especially late gadolinium enhancement imaging, have advanced our ability to better understand and accurately identify fibrosis in the atrial myocardium of atrial fibrillation patients.

According to the nephron number hypothesis, individuals born with kidneys with fewer nephrons would be at increased risk for hypertension and renal disease later in life. Evidence supporting a role for preterm birth itself as a programming risk factor come from observations demonstrating that the degree of prematurity impacts the severity of hypertension or renal dysfunction observed later in life, indicating a dose-response effect of preterm birth. As such, the authors review this effect in the context of consequences for the mother after pregnancy as well as individuals born during premature labor.

This compilation goes on to discuss venous thromboembolism, a spectrum of disease that includes both deep venous thrombosis and pulmonary embolism. Venous thromboembolism affects 950,000 patients every year and is associated with significant morbidity and mortality.

Superior mesenteric artery syndrome is a rare clinical entity resulting in partial or complete duodenal obstruction due to compression of the third part of the duodenum. Symptoms will vary depending on the severity, but can be very debilitating. The authors discuss the diagnosis of this rare condition, as well as treatment options.

Next, the surgical anatomy of the superior mesenteric artery is schematized through a subdivision in three segments, each with a different method for surgical dissection, for a better understanding of its surgical anatomy.

The final chapter focuses on the current development of zebrafish models for the screening for cardiotoxic and cardioprotective agents. The administration of endocrine disruptors, cigarette smoke, acrylamide, phthalates and phosphate, heavy metals, inoculation infectious agent, alcohol, surgery and laser light radiations are the major cause of cardiotoxicity in zebrafish.

Chapter 1 - Atrial fibrillation (AF) is initiated and maintained by triggers and the underlying atrial substrate. Due to these complex associations ablation strategies have become the use of substrate-modifying ablation techniques. However, none of these adjunctive strategies have yielded consistent results. Innovations in cardiac magnetic resonance imaging (MRI) techniques, especially late gadolinium enhancement (LGE) imaging, have advanced our ability to better understand and accurately identify fibrosis in the atrial myocardium of AF patients. It is a potent noninvasive diagnostic tool which allows for follow-up investigations without radiation exposure or risk from an invasive percutaneous procedure. Although, it is difficult to scan patients during AF with LGE-MRI, developments in MRI acquisition strategies like beat-to-beat changes in inversion time and intelligent arrhythmia rejection schemes are likely to improve this difficulty. The consideration of atrial fibrosis for the therapeutic management of AF bears the potential to significantly improve AF understanding and clinical outcomes. Nevertheless, LGE-MRI techniques to assess LA fibrosis still require significant expertise. Further technical improvements and more generalized imaging methods need to be established. There is a wide individual variation in the extent of left atrial fibrosis in patients with AF. Voltage mapping as a tool for describing fibrotic changes is still under investigation. It is dependent on several biological and technological variables, and it still needs to be standardized. The novel multi-atlas-based whole heart segmentation and super-pixel classification-based atrial scarring segmentation have obtained satisfactory accuracy. The combination of patient-specific left atrial and pulmonary geometry model with an objective manual processing atrial scarring segmentation will certainly be beneficial. All ablation strategies beyond PV isolation including fibrosis-guided ablation need to be confirmed and validated with respect to efficacy as well as safety in prospective multicenter randomized clinical studies. The DECAAF II study will probably help to improve the wide adoption of this important imaging tool.

Chapter 2 - Venous thromboembolism (VTE) is a spectrum of disease that includes both deep venous thrombosis (DVT) and pulmonary embolism (PE). VTE affects 950,000 patients every year, including 500,000 new cases of acute DVT. DVT and acute PE are associated with significant morbidity and mortality. For example, every year 60,000 to 100,000 Americans die from VTE/PE, and PE is the third most common cause of cardiovascular death. 10% of PE are fatal within 1 hour, and 5-10% of patients present in shock. Up to 60% of patients with acute DVT will develop post-thrombotic syndrome (PTS).

Chapter 3 - Superior mesenteric artery (SMA) syndrome is a rare clinical entity. It results in partial or complete duodenal obstruction, due to compression of the third part of the duodenum between the superior mesenteric artery and the aorta. This is due to loss of the mesenteric fat pad. It can present acutely, although it is usually has a more insidious onset. Symptoms will vary depending on the severity, but can be very debilitating.

The causes vary, but are usually associated with significant weight loss. It is often diagnosed late, and can require multiple investigations to confirm the diagnosis. Treatment is primarily aimed at increasing weight, but surgical intervention is often required.

The authors discuss the presentation and diagnosis of this rare condition, and treatment options.

Chapter 4 - The superior mesenteric artery (SMA) can be subdivided into three segments for an easier comprehension of its surgical anatomy.

The first segment is the most proximally placed, behind the body of the pancreas; the second is positioned medially to the duodeno-jejunal junction, and the third, the most distal, is located at the base of mesenteries of the transverse colon and of the small bowel. This spatial arrangement involves different surgical approaches.

The dissection of the first segment is the most challenging and requires a surgical approach through the retroperitoneum, medially displacing the left colon and the spleno-pancreatic block. The second segment is approached by mobilizing the duodeno-jejunal junction, and the third, through dissecting at the base of the mesenteries of the transverse colon and of the small bowel.

In case of pancreatic cancer, a secondary involvement of the SMA can be verified through its direct exploration, performed with a Kocher's maneuver in cephalic tumors, or moving down the duodeno-jejunal junction in tumors of the body or of the tail of the pancreas.

Chapter 5 - Over the past decade, zebrafishes have been employed as a key model for various drug screening processes such as cancer, infectious disease, neurodegeneration, pain, dementia, toxicology and so on. This chapter focused on the current development of zebrafish models for the screening for cardiotoxic and cardioprotective agents. Various methods have been employed in the development of cardiotoxicity in zebrafish. The administration or exposure of endocrine disruptors, cigarette smoke, acrylamide, phthalates & phosphate, heavy metals, inoculation infectious agent, alcohol, surgery (cryosection & amputation) and laser light radiations are the major cause of cardiotoxicity in zebrafish. Hence, zebrafishes have been considered as an appropriate tool in the assessment of cardiotoxicity in experimental research and drug discovery process due to numerous advantages over mammalian models. Further, it allows analyzing the variety of cardiovascular and hemodynamic parameters. Therefore, zebrafish can broaden horizons in the field of cardiovascular research.

In: Horizons in World Cardiovascular … ISBN: 978-1-53616-157-1
Editor: Eleanor H. Bennington

Chapter 1

ACCURACY OF LATE GADOLINIUM ENHANCEMENT-MAGNETIC RESONANCE IMAGING IN THE ASSESSMENT OF LEFT ATRIAL MYOCARDIAL FIBROSIS AND SUBSTRATE REMODELING IN PATIENTS WITH ATRIAL FIBRILLATION

***Osmar Antonio Centurión*[1,2,*], *José Carlos Candia*[1], *Laura Beatriz García*[1,2], *Judith María Torales*[1,2], *Orlando Robert Sequeira*[1], *Karina Elizabeth Scavenius*[1,2] and *Luis Marcelo Miño*[1,2]**

[1]Division of Cardiovascular Medicine. Clinic Hospital. Asuncion National University (UNA). San Lorenzo, Paraguay
[2]Department of Health Sciences Investigation. Sanatorio Metropolitano. Fernando de la Mora. Paraguay

[*] Corresponding Author's Email: osmarcenturion@hotmail.com.

Abstract

Atrial fibrillation (AF) is initiated and maintained by triggers and the underlying atrial substrate. Due to these complex associations ablation strategies have become the use of substrate-modifying ablation techniques. However, none of these adjunctive strategies have yielded consistent results. Innovations in cardiac magnetic resonance imaging (MRI) techniques, especially late gadolinium enhancement (LGE) imaging, have advanced our ability to better understand and accurately identify fibrosis in the atrial myocardium of AF patients. It is a potent noninvasive diagnostic tool which allows for follow-up investigations without radiation exposure or risk from an invasive percutaneous procedure. Although, it is difficult to scan patients during AF with LGE-MRI, developments in MRI acquisition strategies like beat-to-beat changes in inversion time and intelligent arrhythmia rejection schemes are likely to improve this difficulty. The consideration of atrial fibrosis for the therapeutic management of AF bears the potential to significantly improve AF understanding and clinical outcomes. Nevertheless, LGE-MRI techniques to assess LA fibrosis still require significant expertise. Further technical improvements and more generalized imaging methods need to be established. There is a wide individual variation in the extent of left atrial fibrosis in patients with AF. Voltage mapping as a tool for describing fibrotic changes is still under investigation. It is dependent on several biological and technological variables, and it still needs to be standardized. The novel multi-atlas-based whole heart segmentation and super-pixel classification-based atrial scarring segmentation have obtained satisfactory accuracy. The combination of patient-specific left atrial and pulmonary geometry model with an objective manual processing atrial scarring segmentation will certainly be beneficial. All ablation strategies beyond PV isolation including fibrosis-guided ablation need to be confirmed and validated with respect to efficacy as well as safety in prospective multicenter randomized clinical studies. The DECAAF II study will probably help to improve the wide adoption of this important imaging tool.

Keywords: atrial fibrillation, cardiac magnetic resonance imaging, 3D electroanatomic mapping, atrial fibrosis, voltage mapping, fractionated atrial electrograms, reentrant rhythms

INTRODUCTION

Fibrotic atrial myocardial tissue is composed of disorganized myocytes and collagen in an expanded extracellular space. There is extensive evidence that atrial wall fibrosis plays a central role in stabilizing the reentrant drivers that initiate and maintain the atrial arrhythmia, specifically atrial fibrillation (AF) [1-4]. Atrial fibrous tissue content and distribution in patients with AF are related not only to AF mechanisms but also to the risk for cardiovascular complications and therapeutic failure [3-5]. Clinical fibrosis imaging promises to provide useful information to guide AF therapy, while a better understanding of how to prevent fibrosis may open up new targets for the development of novel treatment approaches [1-5]. Currently available atrial mapping systems can record electrical activation information, catheter and lesion location, and are capable of tracking catheters in real time. Combining this electrical and navigational information with the explicit three dimensional anatomy of the left atrial chamber and pulmonary veins, should increase the efficacy of atrial fibrillation ablation procedures.

In the myocardial tissue, fibroblasts are small, spindle-shaped cells that comprise the structure of the extracellular matrix. Although fibroblasts constitute up to 75% of cardiac cells by number, they consist only 10% to 15% by mass [6]. Fibroblasts proliferate and differentiate into a secretory but non-proliferative phenotype called the myofibroblast when activated by certain pro-fibrotic stimuli. The source of both latter cells in remodeled myocardium is not clearly understood, with evidence for contributions from resident fibroblasts, bone marrow–derived cells, endothelial cells, perivascular cells, and pericytes [7]. The fibrotic process is a complex one that involves increased production and activity of a variety of extracellular matrix proteins secreted by fibroblasts. These proteins include fibronectin, procollagen, collagen cross-linking agents such as lysyl oxidase, and enzymes such as matrix metalloproteinases and tissue-inhibitors of matrix metalloproteinases [6, 7].

Atrial fibrosis can be considered to consist of 2 principal types, namely reactive and reparative fibrosis [8-10]. First, in reactive or interstitial fibrosis there is proliferation of fibroblast and differentiation to the secretory myofibroblast phenotype, and accumulation of collagen in the perivascular space and the perimysium surrounding cardiac muscle bundles. Second, reparative or replacement fibrosis occurs when fibrous tissue replaces zones of dead muscle cells like myocardial infarction scar [7, 9]. This type of atrial fibrosis may be largely irreversible, and is associated with extensive cell death and regions of fibrosis that interrupt the muscle bundles producing clear longitudinal conduction barriers [11, 12]. These different types of fibrosis are not necessarily mutually exclusive, and many patients may well have combinations of interstitial and replacement fibrosis in the atria. Pro-fibrotic signaling involves a complex set of interacting pathways and molecular signaling systems [13-16]. Major pro-fibrotic cell membrane receptors include those for connective tissue growth factor, angiotensin-II type 1 receptors, platelet derived growth factor, and transforming growth factor-beta. Inflammation and its many associated cytokines and cellular mediators are also highly effective in releasing and activating pro-fibrotic molecules and causing fibrosis [17-21].

Myocardial cells and fibroblasts are able to develop low-resistance electric junctions and modulate each other's electrical activity in co-cultured systems [22, 23]. The degree of interaction and its significance depends on the number of fibroblasts coupled to each myocardial cell and the degree of coupling, as well as, the relative size of the myocardial cells to fibroblasts size [24-27]. Significant coupling at the cardiomyocyte-fibroblast junction can enhance phase 4-depolarization and promote ectopic beats [6] and can also slow impulse conduction and promote the development of re-entrant arrhythmias especially AF [23]. Therefore, it is our intention to analyze the accuracy of late gadolinium enhancement-magnetic resonance imaging in the assessment of left atrial myocardial fibrosis and substrate remodeling in patients with atrial fibrillation.

Mechanisms and Physiopathology of Atrial Fibrosis

It was observed that myocardial fibrosis may result from inflammation, as well as, microvascular ischemia and reactive or reparative patterns may be seen in human and animal experimental histological studies [28-38]. The mechanisms for myocardial fibrosis are undoubtedly multi-factorial. It is the resultant of a combination of several factors including genetic predisposition, exposure to toxins and pathogens, microvascular ischemia, and abnormal modulation of immune and metabolic responses. Mechanical stretch is also an important fibroblast activator and stimulus to fibrosis [17]. Functional mitral regurgitation and rapid left atrial dilatation are common consequences of atrial fibrosis-associated AF [18], and atrial stretch is likely a central pro-fibrotic stimulus in many study models. Collagen synthesis begins in the endoplasmic reticulum with the production of pro-collagen which is a collagen precursor [19-21]. Type I collagen, which constitutes 80% to 90% of collagen in fibrous tissue, is produced from pro-collagen alpha 1 and alpha 2 chains. Each procollagen-1 molecule consists of two alpha 1 chains and one alpha 2 chain, which form a central coiled alpha helix with procollagen C-terminal proteinase and procollagen N-terminal proteinase. Procollagen-3 consists of three procollagen-3 alpha chains. Procollagen is secreted from the cell into the extracellular space and mature collagen molecules are formed via terminal-terminal self-assembly. The final step in collagen formation is oxidative cross-linking by lysyl oxidase and related lysyl oxidase–like enzymes [19-21]. Although a wide range of proteins are expressed in the extracellular matrix and are involved in the pro-fibrotic response, relatively little is known about their roles in atrial fibrosis and about whether manipulating their expression or function can be useful in the therapeutic management.

It was demonstrated in histopathologic studies the existence of significant interstitial replacement and perivascular fibrosis in the myocardium (Figure 1) [39-41]. These fibrous tissues in ischemic or non-ischemic substrate may enhance the non-uniform anisotropy leading to delayed conduction and unidirectional conduction block generating reentrant circuits and cardiac arrhythmias [42-45]. It was also shown that increased myocardial fibrosis was the cause for non-uniform anisotropic propagation and fractionated electrograms [46-48]. It was demonstrated that most of the new reentrant wave fronts were initiated by epicardial breakthrough, which was followed by a line of conduction block parallel to the epicardial fiber orientation. This was accomplished in nicely done studies performed with explanted hearts supported by Langendorff perfusion techniques and computerized mapping system [49]. These findings suggest the importance of increased fibrosis, and increased tissue anisotropy in the initiation of reentry. Anisotropic conduction plays an important role in the development of various types of atrial and ventricular arrhythmias [50-60].

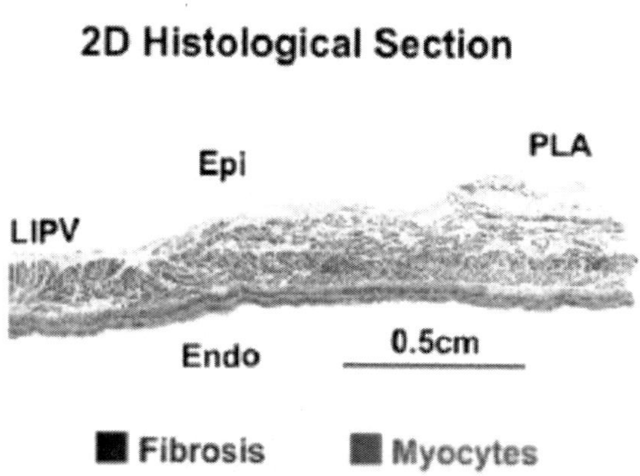

Figure 1. Visualization of transmural fibrosis by histology. 2-dimensional (2D) histology sections stained by Masson's trichrome. Endo: Endocardium. Epi: Epicardium. LIPV: Left inferior pulmonary vein. PLA: Posterior left atrium. Reprinted with permission from Zhao J, Hansen BJ, Wang Y, Csepe TA, Sul LV, Tang A, et al. Three-dimensional Integrated Functional, Structural, and Computational Mapping to Define the Structural "Fingerprints" of Heart-Specific Atrial Fibrillation Drivers in Human Heart *Ex Vivo*. J Am Heart Assoc. 2017; 6: e005922. DOI: 10.1161/JAHA.117.005922.

Dillon SM et al. [61] showed that anisotropic conduction and block may result from muscle fiber separation by connective tissue in the epicardial border zone. It was also reported that the greater incidence of atrial arrhythmias with age may be caused by the development of extensive collagenous septa dividing the myocardial fibers [43]. Interstitial fibrosis and broad bands of scarring was another structural complexity characteristic of slow conduction and delayed depolarization activation [62, 63]. An increase of fibrous tissues between the muscle fibers and bundles may enhance non-uniform anisotropy and promote electrical uncoupling [42, 43]. In this context, impulse propagation and depolarization through atrial tissue may fail in the transverse direction but not in the longitudinal propagation, resulting in unidirectional conduction block [64-66]. Therefore, the distal zone to the line of block may be activated by the slowly propagating transverse wave front allowing a longer delay for the proximal fibers to regain excitability to develop reentry and AF.

The mechanism and clinical implications of myocardial fibrosis has been extensively studied in the ventricular myocardium [67-80]. Several studies that analyzed the ventricular arrhythmia substrate found that myocardial fibrosis plays an important role in the genesis of ventricular arrhythmias [81-90]. The arrhythmogenic substrate in the ventricular myocardium and its role in the pathophysiology of ventricular arrhythmias and sudden cardiac death have been investigated, and it is thought to have a number of different pathways and several contributing mechanisms. Therefore, the evaluation of ventricular fibrosis by LGE-MRI has been suggested as an indicator for sudden cardiac death risk stratification [91-99]. The left ventricular remodeling process that experience patients with heart failure is characterized by changes in the extracellular matrix, including the formation of fibrotic tissue [100-102]. The surrounding zone of the area of fibrosis is a heterogeneous medium, where tissue with different levels of fibrosis coexists, resulting in both viable and nonviable myocardium [102]. This ventricular myocardial fibrosis may constitute a substrate for ventricular tachycardia, where slow and heterogeneous conduction may favor the genesis of reentry mechanism increasing the chance to develop malignant ventricular arrhythmias [102-105]. It was clearly demonstrated in clinical studies that the finding of myocardial fibrosis by cardiac MRI is associated with a poor prognosis in HF patients, and it is associated to the pathogenesis of sustained ventricular tachycardia and ventricular fibrillation [106-110]. These zones of myocardial fibrosis consist of areas of late gadolinium enhancement visualized on cardiac MRI (Figure 2). These LGE-MRI areas are present in nearly 30% of patients with heart failure [111-113]. The presence of mid-wall fibrosis is utilized as indicator to individualize patients at high risk of arrhythmic events in heart failure [85-87]. Most of the studies analyzing the scar, total LGE or gray-zone extent, demonstrated a statistically significant relation effect with the risk of ventricular tachycardia. Larger and more heterogeneous scars were found to have higher probabilities of ventricular arrhythmias during the follow-up period [86-90]. Nevertheless, further studies with larger populations are necessary to assess the actual performance of the gray-zone in risk stratification. In addition, there is a necessity for optimization of gray-zone detection protocols since they involve complex and operator-dependent techniques [104].

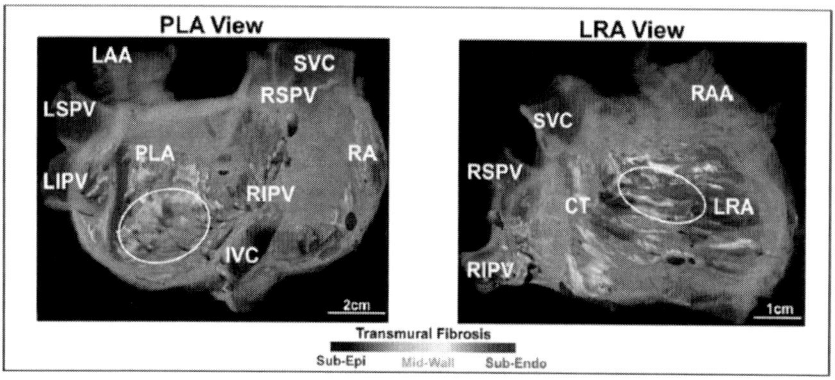

Figure 2. Transmural fibrosis of the intact human atria. Three-dimensional (3D) fibrosis distribution across the whole human atria. Fibrosis distribution in atrial volume visualized transmurally. Fibrosis transmurality is displayed in the PLA and LRA, respectively. The white ovals indicate the locations of AF driver regions defined by optical mapping. CT: crista terminalis. Endo: endocardium; Epi: epicardium. IVC/SVC: inferior/superior vena cava. LA/RA: left/right atrium. LAA/RAA: left/right atrial appendage. LRA: lateral right atrium. LSPV/LIPV/RSPV/RIPV: left superior/left inferior/right superior/right inferior pulmonary vein. PLA: posterior left atrium. Reprinted with permission from Zhao J, Hansen BJ, Wang Y, Csepe TA, Sul LV, Tang A, et al. Three-dimensional Integrated Functional, Structural, and Computational Mapping to Define the Structural "Fingerprints" of Heart-Specific Atrial Fibrillation Drivers in Human Heart *Ex Vivo*. J Am Heart Assoc. 2017; 6: e005922. DOI: 10.1161/JAHA.117.005922.

Fibrotic changes in the atrial myocardium have been shown to be highly associated to the initiation and maintenance AF [114-118]. According to the European Society of Cardiology guidelines [119] and a recently published consensus document on atrial cardiomyopathy [120], the understanding of AF is changing from a sole rhythm disturbance toward the concept of a combined rhythm plus atrial cardiomyopathy phenomenon that is well interconnected. The expert consensus paper from the EHRA/HRS/APHRS/SOLAECE on atrial cardiomyopathies: definition, characterization, and clinical implication, characterizes this atrial cardiomyopathy as "any complex of structural, architectural, contractile or electro-physiological changes affecting the atria with the potential to produce clinically-relevant manifestations" [120]. "AF begets AF", this concept of the self-perpetuation of AF by structural remodeling is well established in experimental animal models [114]. For example, studies performed in goats have shown that high-frequency atrial pacing leads to atrial remodeling with a de-differentiation of atrial muscle cells to a more fetal phenotype [115]. *In vitro* data suggest a profound cardiomyocyte–fibroblast interaction regulating the myofibroblast function that can result in an increase in atrial interstitial fibrosis [116]. These atrial fibrotic changes have been shown to maintain AF and to increase its burden [117, 118]. Several observations obtained by auxiliary diagnostic methods in recent years have led to new mechanistic insights in AF. Imaging atrial fibrosis using enhanced LGE-MRI may be an option to identify the patients at risk for AF before the initiation of the arrhythmia. Cochet et al. [121] demonstrated significant structural changes in the atria of non-AF individuals. Mahnkopf et al. [122] stated that this atrial myopathy may be a precursor for the development of AF by demonstrating that fibrotic atrial alterations are already present in the early stages of AF. In order to monitor the effect of invasive approaches on structural remodeling, the results of studies with LGE-MRI suggest a potential regression of structural alterations, which is best when AF ablation is performed in early Utah stages [123]. Those mechanistic insights may provide the hypothesis for future cohort and investigational studies assessing progression and reversibility of atrial fibrotic remodeling by interventions.

Moe GK, et al. [124-126] suggested that if a wave front progresses through tissue that is irregularly excitable, it will be irregularly refracted traveling at non-uniform velocities over non-uniform paths, leaving non-uniform tissue in their wake. Therefore, they stated that non-uniformity would increase the degree of fractionation of wave fronts. In the multiple wavelet hypothesis of atrial fibrillation, Moe GK et al. suggested that the persistence of fibrillation depends upon the average total number of wavelets that the tissue can support. Any factor that increases the average number of wavelets will tend to perpetuate the arrhythmia. In addition, if the conduction velocity is slowed, a given mass of atrial tissue can support a greater mean number of wavelets. They hypothesized that AF was due to functional reentry of multiple wavelets, rather than to rapidly firing ectopic foci. Reentry, either functional or anatomic, has several pre-requisites. In the first place, there should be an atrial substrate allowing for unidirectional block, with concomitant conduction over a discreet limb of the circuit. In the second place, the wavelength of the depolarization during tachycardia must fit in the excitable, repolarized tissue available. The wavelength of the depolarization is defined by the product of conduction velocity and refractory period. Conditions that reduce the wavelength of depolarized tissue, either by shortening atrial effective refractory period and/or reducing atrial conduction velocity, are likely to contribute to sustained atrial rhythms. Allessie MA, et al. confirmed the multiple wavelet hypotheses put forth by Gordon Moe [127-129]. AF induced by rapid pacing was shown to shorten atrial refractory periods, leading to ever-increasing predisposition for AF induction and maintenance and demonstrating the observation that AF begets AF [127]. In his initial study of pacing-induced AF in goats, Allessie MA, et al. did not find significant changes in atrial conduction velocity. However, subsequent studies performed by other researchers have found that conduction velocity in atrial tissue prone to sustained fibrillation is significantly compromised [130]. There is likely a number of factors that contribute to deranged activation propagation in diseased atrial tissue. These include alterations in gap junction protein expression [131-136], attendant changes in myocyte coupling, and the development of interstitial fibrosis and atrial scarring [130]. All of these factors reduce conduction velocity, generate regions of anisotropic conduction and lines of frank conduction block, and thus contribute to the initiation and maintenance of functional atrial reentry.

The decision to invasively treat an AF patient is currently based on symptoms, temporal behavior of the arrhythmia, age, and comorbidities associated with the arrhythmia [118, 137]. Since enhanced LGE-MRI atrial fibrosis has been shown to be a powerful predictor for clinical outcome when correcting for other confounding factors, it may successfully guide the therapeutic decision making (Figure 3) [138]. For patients with Utah classes III/IV with diffuse and extensive fibrosis, a conventional, noninvasive approach should be considered because the potential for long-term freedom from AF is very low after AF catheter ablation (Figure 4) [139-142]. Moreover, pre-ablation LGE-MRI can also help in counseling patients about the expected outcome of catheter ablation and also alternative treatment options.

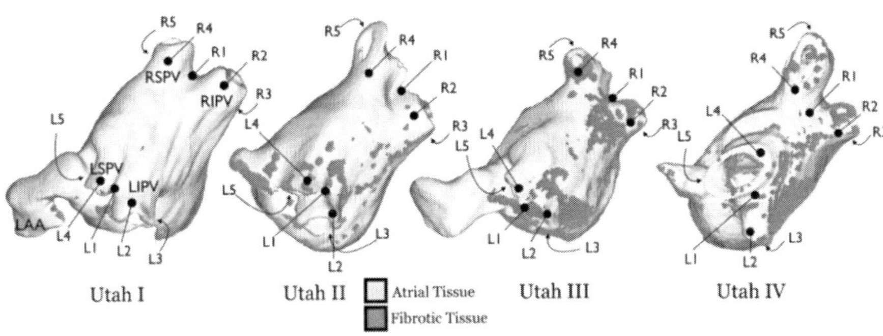

Figure 3. Patient-specific distributions of LA fibrosis for substrates Utah stages I—IV. Pacing locations in the left PVs (L1–L5) and right PVs (R1–R5) are indicated for each substrate. Anatomical locations for the left superior PV (LSPV), left inferior PV (LIPV), right superior PV (RSPV), right inferior PV (RIPV), and LA appendage (LAA) are indicated in the left-most substrate; all substrates are presented in identical orientations. Reprinted with permission from McDowell KS, Zahid S, Vadakkumpadan F, Blauer J, MacLeod RS, Trayanova NA. Virtual Electrophysiological Study of Atrial Fibrillation in Fibrotic Remodeling. PLoS ONE 2015; 10(2): e0117110. doi:10.1371/journal.pone.0117110.

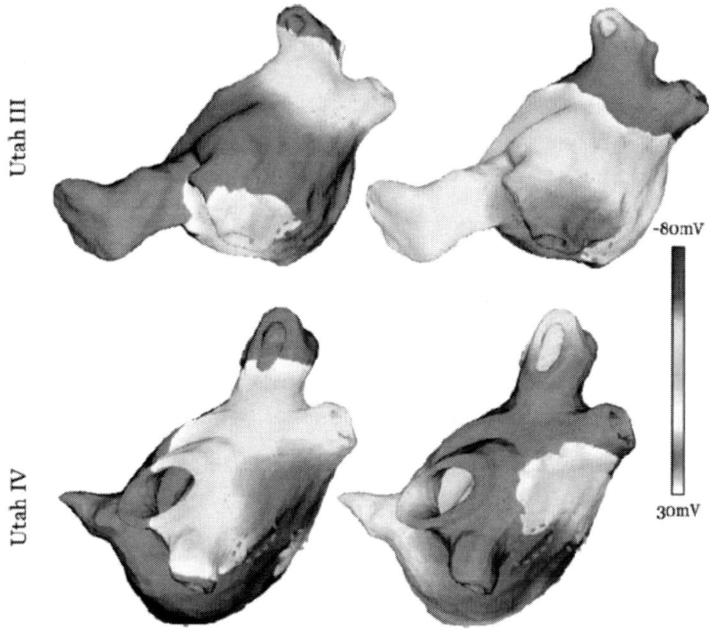

Figure 4. Epicardial transmembrane potential maps at two time instants in atrial models Utah III (top row) and Utah IV (bottom row) demonstrating an instant location of the phase singularity at the time instant of the transmembrane potential map, as well as the outline of the confined region of precession of the persistent phase singularities. Reprinted with permission from McDowell KS, Zahid S, Vadakkumpadan F, Blauer J, MacLeod RS, Trayanova NA. Virtual Electrophysiological Study of Atrial Fibrillation in Fibrotic Remodeling. PLoS ONE 2015; 10(2): e0117110. doi:10.1371/journal.pone.0117110.

Treatment approaches and therapeutic measurements to reduce the risk for AF, such as blood pressure control, reducing alcohol intake, moderate exercise, and optimization of other comorbidities, have already been shown to be effective in certain groups of patients. These clinical approaches and therapeutic measures may decrease the AF development by reducing the atrial fibrotic burden [119, 142, 143]. The possibility to visualize and quantify an atrial substrate by LGE-MRI offers the chance to determine the effect of upstream interventions by documentation of progression or reversal of atrial remodeling. Atrial fibrosis assessment may also have the potential to further clarify the role of antiarrhythmic effects of non-antiarrhythmic drugs in terms of upstream therapy, as already suggested for angiotensin-converting enzyme inhibitors [144, 145]. Proper patient selection is mandatory to investigate several drugs agent beneficial effects in specific subgroups of patients with mild early fibrosis in whom AF is very likely to develop.

There is increasing evidence for an association of AF, atrial fibrosis, and ischemic cerebrovascular accidents. Stroke due to arterial embolism of cardiac origin is a dreadful complication. Fibrosis detected using LGE-MRI has been demonstrated to be associated with stroke [146]. It was also demonstrated that pre-ablation fibrosis burden is a significant risk factor for the presence of spontaneous echo contrast in transesophageal echocardiography. This latter finding adds additional predictive power to already establish risk scores [137, 147, 148]. On the other hand, there are certain disagreement on the association of AF and Stroke. The ASSERT Trial showed that stroke events had only a very poor correlation to the time of AF episodes [149]. In addition, it was shown that the risk of stroke might be independently associated with structural fibrotic remodeling in the absence of AF in patients with a rare autosomal recessive disease, namely, atrial dilated cardiomyopathy [150]. Further considerations suggest a potential underlying pro-coagulative state, mediated by proteinase activated receptor signaling pathways, which on the one hand might predispose to thromboembolic events and on the other hand contribute to atrial fibrosis [151]. With these findings into consideration, the risk of stroke in AF may be considered as a continuum in which cumulative risk factors have to be assessed in details, and the additional value of fibrosis assessment has to be further investigated in prospective controlled trials [152].

AF has clear associations with other common entities. The association between AF and heart failure was initially described more than 100 years ago [153]. The actual prevalence of AF in heart failure is estimated to be as high as 13% to 27%, and up to 40% in advanced heart failure [154]. AF may be both the cause and consequence of heart failure, and in most cases, the causal relationship between AF and heart failure may be driven by ventricular dysfunction which promotes atrial wall fibrosis perpetuating AF [155-159]. It was clearly shown that depressed LV energetics remain unaltered, independent from restoration of sinus rhythm, suggesting a primary ventricular cause. Atrial fibrosis is considered a key player in the development of AF on the basis of heart failure [159-161]. Another interesting study using LGE-MRI [162] showed that AF patients with heart failure present with a higher degree of atrial fibrosis, further highlighting a causal relationship between LV dysfunction and atrial structural remodeling leading to AF initiation and maintenance. Since there is only little information on human studies assessing the role of atrial fibrosis in the setting of heart failure, further research is warranted.

Imaging studies with enhanced LGE-MRI should be considered to analyze left atrial fibrosis and its progression before and after initial and repeat AF catheter ablation [163-165]. These studies provide promising results to visualize the temporal behavior of atrial fibrosis after ablation by subtracting post-ablation scarring from the total extent of initial fibrotic atrial tissue. It was demonstrated that patients without AF recurrence after catheter ablation showed a significant reduction in LA fibrosis burden in follow-up LGE-MRI studies [165]. Atrial fibrosis reflects the hallmark of structural remodeling of the atrium, hence, assessment of changes of fibrotic alterations may shed some light and give new insights into AF treatment strategies in case of AF recurrence after catheter ablation [136, 163-166]. Enhanced LGE-MRI improves our understanding of the causal and temporal relationship of electrical and structural remodeling in the natural course of AF. Since fibrotic tissue would yield a low voltage signal, voltage mapping by sampling electrical signals from atrial tissue is the gold standard to assess and stage the extent of atrial fibrosis [167]. Almost 20 years ago, Callans DJ, et al. [168] already described a correlation between electroanatomic properties and histopathological findings of fibrotic alterations in porcine animal models. Jadidi AS, et al. [169] reported a correlation of MRI data and electrophysiological properties describing lower bipolar voltage in fibrotic areas compared with non-fibrotic tissue. In this context, we should be cautions and bear in mind that slow conduction induced by functional alterations, namely, connexin changes can mimic low voltage without being related to fibrotic remodeling [170].

Arbitrary thresholds to define fibrotic areas have been established in clinical practice during the beginning of 3D electroanatomic mapping studies. Since then a bipolar voltage ≤ 0.05 mV has been considered as atrial scar on the basis of baseline noise in those early electroanatomic mapping studies [171-173]. The first point-by-point comparison of fibrosis, assessed by LGE-MRI, and endocardial voltage demonstrating that increasing levels of LGE correlate with lower voltages was provided only five years ago [172]. Enhanced LGE-MRI levels of 5 standard deviation above blood pool were correlated to 0.38 ± 0.28 mV, indicating that 0.05 mV as an arbitrary threshold might underestimate the extent of fibrotic areas [172, 169]. In addition, since Harrison et al. [171], reported that ablation-induced scarring reveals a voltage of 0.3 to 0.6 mV, a threshold of ≤0.05 could significantly underestimate the extent of ablation injury. These are very interesting data that we have to be considered in order to set adequate values of normality. This work [171] provided the first histopathological validation of enhanced LGE-MRI and endocardial voltage mapping for definition of atrial scarring with acute and chronic ablation injury by providing signal intensity thresholds for both ablation types. Therefore, patient-specific cutoff voltage values for fibrosis have to be well-established, and more histopathological validation studies for atrial fibrosis have to be done. The multiple diagnostic auxiliary methods necessary to perform the best in the therapeutic guidance of AF management shows how complex the therapeutic management of AF is. The necessity to combine various imaging modalities like fluoroscopy, 3D electroanatomic mapping, enhanced LGE-MRI, and intracardiac echocardiography guidance, to optimize the results of AF ablation implies the technical difficulties in performing this therapeutic approach. On the other hand, the necessity to combine different AF ablation techniques, namely, circumferential, linear, and targeted ablation of complex fractionated electrograms, in order to improve the success rate demonstrates the complexity of the electrophysiological substrate in atrial fibrillation. Currently, enhanced LGE-MRI offers the option to assess atrial structure in 3D in one hand, and in the other, 3D electroanatomic mapping with endocardial surface as provided by voltage mapping are able to reliably identify the location and transmural extent of fibrotic changes. Currently, other methods to assess structural changes are being investigated. Transthoracic echocardiography studies demonstrated that 3D speckle tracking offers the chance to obtain information on mechanical and substrate abnormalities [136, 174].

The DECAAF II is an ongoing prospective, randomized, multi-center trial of patients with persistent Atrial Fibrillation (AF) and presence of atrial fibrosis. The lead investigator is Dr. Nassir Marrouche from Utah University. Enrollment is currently underway for this study, and as of December 19, 2018, there were 41 sites enrolling patients. By the end of January 2019, it is expect 2 additional sites to be enrolling. Currently there are 766 patients enrolled in the study. This ongoing DECAAF II trial will probably generate additional insights into the role of atrial fibrosis as a potential target for catheter ablation of AF. This additional information could help to improve our understanding of the underlying mechanisms driving AF, and could serve as a basis for establishing novel ablation approaches, namely, ablation of rotational activity or focal triggers.

Atrial Fibrosis and Prolonged and Fractionated Atrial Electrograms

Details and the precise mechanism by which fibrosis contributes to the origination and maintenance of AF is not fully understood. AF initiation and maintenance depends on interplay between triggers and substrate. Traditionally, triggers are thought to be localized to the PV ostia, though increase in fibrosis may give rise to new, non-PV localized trigger sites, namely, the crista terminalis, ligament of Marshal, Bachman´s bundle, and also near the cava veins. Increased fibrosis almost certainly changes the conduction properties of the tissue activated by triggered beats, such that fibrosis is an important contributor to AF maintenance. Animal models of tachycardia-mediated cardiomyopathy suggest that regions of left atrial fibrosis result in increased conduction heterogeneity through the left atrium, with both large patches of fibrosis and pulmonary vein ostia serving as anchors reentrant circuits and impediments to conduction that result in delays, and lines of block [175-180].

Studies performed with mathematical modeling work suggest that fibroblast proliferation may contribute to the generation of prolonged and fractionated electrograms in humans [181]. In addition, fibroblast ion-channel remodeling might significantly alter the electrophysiological properties and the maintaining and persistence of AF [182]. It still remains unknown whether the extent to which the effects of fibrosis on atrial conduction are due to the production of collagen that separates cardiomyocytes and physically uncouples them [183-185], or to the proliferation of fibroblasts that couple to cardiomyocytes and electrically load them [186]. There is indirect evidence supporting a role for fibroblast-cardiomyocyte interactions on ventricular conduction after myocardial infarction [187], but it remains uncertain whether there are sufficient numbers of fibroblasts that are sufficiently well coupled to cardiomyocytes to alter atrial conduction *in vivo* myocardial tissue.

There is increasing evidence of atrial fibrosis as an atrial structural substrate for the genesis of atrial arrhythmias. Histopathological evidence of extensive fibrosis of the sinoatrial node associated with fiber degeneration and increased fibrosis of atrial myocardium in the approaches to the sinus node and internodal tracts has been clearly demonstrated in patients with sinus node dysfunction and atrial fibrillation [188]. When an atrial depolarization traverses an atrial structural substrate with extensive fibrosis, the depolarization wave suffers of conduction slowing and fractionation. This produces abnormal atrial electrograms (AAE) that can be recorded during sinus rhythm by atrial endocardial catheter mapping (Figure 5). Fractionated electrograms were recorded from areas of human atrial muscle where fibrous tissue separated the muscle fibers from each other [189]. In a previous report we demonstrated in patients with sinus node dysfunction but without tachyarrhythmias, that AAE were mostly localized in the high right atrium in the vicinity of the sinus node, suggesting a more localized electrophysiological abnormality [190]. On the other hand, in patients with sinus node dysfunction and paroxysmal AF, AAE were rather widely distributed within the right atrium, suggesting a more diffuse electrophysiological abnormality of the atrial muscle [190].

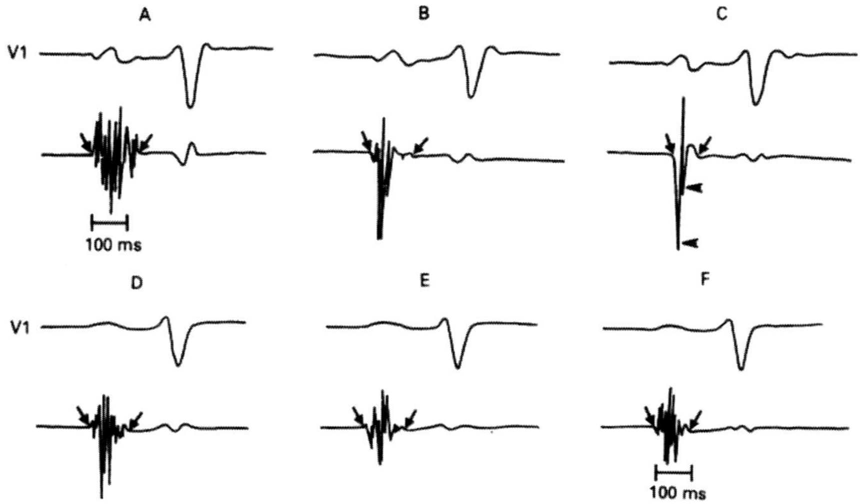

Figure 5. Six atrial electrograms recorded at different right atrial sites in two patients with Sinus Node Dysfunction (A, B, and C in a SND patient with Rubenstein Type I and II; D, E, and F in a SND patient with Rubenstein Type III with Atrial Fibrillation). Diagonal arrows represent the onset and offset of local electrical activity and horizontal arrows the downward deflections. Reprinted with permission from Centurión OA, Fukatani M, Konoe A, Tanigawa M, Shimizu A, Isomoto S y col. Different distribution of abnormal endocardial electrogram within the right atrium in patients with sick sinus syndrome. Br Heart J 1992; 68: 596-600.

It was shown that AAE indicate areas of altered anatomy and conduction where reentry is likely to develop. Moreover, patients with sinus node dysfunction and AF have histologically proven fibrosis and degenerative lesions of the atrium walls. Therefore, with these facts in mind, Centurión OA et al. [191] attempted to relate the findings of AAE to atrial conduction defects and induced or spontaneous episodes of atrial fibrillation in patients with sick sinus node dysfunction. In this context, we have found a significantly longer conduction time of sinus impulses in our sinus node dysfunction patients who possess AAE within the right atrium, as compared to those patients with sinus node dysfunction who do not have AAE. In addition, no significant difference was observed in the functional or effective refractory periods of the atrium among patients with or without AAE. Leier et al. [192] reported a significant prolongation of the mean right intra-atrial conduction time at 50 ms, and the mean interatrial conduction time at 92 ms in 21 patients with atrial flutter. In our study [191] the mean intra-atrial (54 ms) and the mean interatrial (100 ms) conduction time of sinus impulses were significantly longer in the AAE (+) Group. Therefore, there is a greater conduction time in patients with AAE. This prolongation in conduction time of sinus impulses through a diseased atrial muscle may be related to a lengthening of the pathway to be traversed and/or slowing of conduction velocity. Our data suggest that the atrial conduction defects, rather than a short effective refractory period, appear to account for the significantly greater propensity of the AAE (+) sinus node dysfunction patients to develop atrial fibrillation [191].

Mary-Rabine L, et al. [193] studying the relationship of human atrial cellular electrophysiology to clinical function and ultrastructure observed that when depressed conduction was manifested in recordings from human atrial muscle the ultrastructure was usually abnormal. Areas of poorly coupled fibers in diseased atrial myocardium with progressive fibrosis and degenerative changes may lead to abnormal electrophysiological characteristics. Connective tissue septa encircling muscle fiber groups reflect sites where electrical coupling between adjacent fibers is difficult to occur. The microarchitecture and anisotropic characteristics of the atrial myocardium may play an important role in reentrant rhythms by causing inhomogeneous and discontinuous propagation of the atrial impulse [191].

Spach MS, et al. [194] observed in muscle bundles with non-uniform anisotropic properties that when propagation occurs in the transverse direction, the waveform is irregular or fractionated due to superimposed small rapid deflections. Structural inhomogeneity or local differences in electrophysiological or ultrastructural properties are considered to play a major role in the initiation of reentrant circuits due to the increased likelihood of unidirectional block of the premature impulse [194-196]. Fibrosis and particularly fibro-fatty infiltration of the atrial myocardium are major determinants for AF and its progression is responsible for increased myocardial stiffness and poor clinical outcome [197-199]. A relationship between impaired atrial strain and fibro-fatty atrial wall infiltration has been demonstrated *in vivo* by MRI [199]. Subsequently, accurately quantifying the amount of adipose tissue and fibrotic remodeling of the human atria is thus a crucial issue. Histology is the gold standard method to quantify myocardial adipose tissue and fibrotic components within the left atrial wall *ex vivo* at the microscopic level. MRI T1 mapping enables quantification of the myocardial signal directly on a standard scale. It has generated great interest since it allows *in vivo* quantitative myocardial tissue characterization non-invasively [200-202], potentially alleviating the need for biopsy. Indeed, at a macroscopic level, native T1 values, although non-specific, have been found to be sensitive markers of the presence and severity of disease [203-205]. The left atrial wall is very thin, only measuring 2 mm. Therefore, it is very challenging to reliably measure T1 values within the left atrial wall without being subject to partial volume effects [206]. Few attempts with T1 mapping techniques have been made to quantify the degree of left atrial myocardial fibrosis noninvasively [207]. However, similar to late gadolinium enhancement of the left atrial wall, whether such MRI measurements exclusively reflect fibrosis is being debated [208, 209].

Atrial fibrosis is not only associated to longer intra-atrial and interatrial conduction times but also with longer P Wave duration. Hordof AJ, et al. [210] found a statistical association between the low resting membrane potential and a prolonged P Wave duration. Josephson ME, et al. [211] reported that a prolonged interatrial conduction time was significantly related to abnormal P Wave morphology. Neither left atrial size nor atrial pressure overload was found to correlate well with abnormal P Wave morphology [211-213]. We have found that patients with sinus node dysfunction who have AAE possess significantly longer P Wave duration and PA intervals than those patients with sinus node dysfunction who do not possess AAE within the right atrium during sinus rhythm [191]. When a single premature atrial stimulation is introduced with a critical timing close to the effective refractory period, some of the extrastimuli may elicit a significant intra-atrial and interatrial conduction delay facilitating AF development. This slow conduction of atrial premature impulses during incomplete recovery of excitability appears to be a major predisposing factor to reentry. Simpson RJ Jr, et al. [214] found a significant correlation between the history of primary atrial tachyarrhythmia and the maximum increase in atrial conduction time of early cycle premature beats. Therefore, they stated that intra-atrial and interatrial conduction delay should be considered as risk factors for atrial tachyarrhythmia. Slowing of the conduction time of atrial premature beats may also explain why early premature beats are more likely to induce AF than later premature beats [215]. Centurión OA, et al. [191] demonstrated that the incidence of induced and spontaneous atrial fibrillation was significantly higher in the AAE (+) sinus node dysfunction patients than that in the sinus node dysfunction patients who do not possess AAE. Abnormal atrial electrograms showed a good specificity and positive predictive accuracy in evaluating inducible and spontaneous atrial fibrillation. However, the sensitivity and negative predictive accuracy was rather lower. Abnormal atrial electrograms were also found to be a relatively useful marker in discriminating patients with severe sinus node disease from those with milder sinus node disease, and in separating patients with more extensive atrial electrical disease who are more likely to have inducible atrial fibrillation from others. We demonstrated that patients with sinus node dysfunction who possessed abnormal atrial electrograms in sinus rhythm had greater atrial conduction defects, wider P wave duration, and a significantly higher incidence of induction of sustained atrial fibrillation [191]. Since abnormal atrial electrograms reflect slow conduction through non-uniform anisotropic atrial muscle, it follows that a greater number of wavelets may be generated and atrial fibrillation would be more likely to be sustained, a fact that is in accordance with our results [191]. Abnormal atrial electrograms may reflect inhomogeneous local electrical activity related to a delayed and non-uniform anisotropic conduction through a diseased atrial muscle. When atrial walls are markedly altered and distorted by fibrosis, the propagating depolarization wave is required to change direction frequently with respect to fiber orientation, creating sites for potential block leading to reentrant arrhythmias. The potential clinical significance is that detection of abnormal atrial electrograms during sinus rhythm in patients with sinus node dysfunction may help to identify those with greater atrial conduction defects and higher incidence of induced and spontaneous episodes of atrial fibrillation.

Since atrial fibrosis plays an important role in the genesis of AF, suppressing fibrosis to prevent AF may be an interesting therapeutic approach. This latter notion was supported experimentally nearly two decades ago [216] and is accepted as a promising potential approach for the development of innovative therapies [217]. There are several signaling systems that could theoretically be targeted to prevent fibrosis. The renin-angiotensin system was the first target for which inhibition was shown experimentally to prevent atrial fibrosis and thereby to ameliorate the AF substrate [216]. From that time on subsequent experimental studies and clinical research have demonstrated the potential to prevent fibrosis through several signaling pathway targets, including TGF-b, inflammatory mediators, heat-shock proteins [217], JAK-STAT signaling [218], miRNAs [219-221], TRP channels [222], and peroxisome proliferator-activated receptor–gamma [223]. Whether some of these specific targets are practical and effective in the clinical setting remains to be determined in clinical trials. Clinical studies have already provided supportive data for the potential value of such upstream therapy for primary prevention of AF, particularly with renin-angiotensin-aldosterone system targeting. However, the results have been less supportive for secondary prevention of AF [224].

In 1982 Goldman MR et al. [225] performed an experimental study to quantify myocardial infarction with contrast-enhanced magnetic resonance imaging [MRI] in excised canine hearts. The clinical application and implications of this pioneering study have multiplied and proliferated due to technical advancement and increasing understanding of cardiac pathophysiology [226-228]. Two years later, gadolinium-based contrast agents were introduced in the diagnostic methodology which constituted a milestone in cardiac imaging [228]. Although it was initially intended to assess ventricular myocardium in the setting of acute and chronic myocardial infarction [227], late gadolinium enhancement (LGE) MRI has recently emerged as a promising tool for assessment of structural alterations of the atrial wall [229]. Atrial fibrosis is a common pathophysiological contributor to initiation and maintenance of atrial arrhythmias and especially

AF. Therefore, including atrial fibrosis imaging with enhanced LGE-MRI into the diagnosis, monitoring, and treatment of AF may be crucial for diagnostic improvements and clinical outcomes, as well as, a better understanding of disease progression [230]. In the context of AF catheter ablation, atrial assessment with LGE-MRI aims at increasing success rates and minimizing cardiovascular complications.

USE OF ENHANCED LGE-MRI FOR IMAGING OF ATRIAL FIBROSIS

LGE-MRI with extracellular gadolinium-based contrast is based on a delayed contrast wash-in and wash-out in myocardial tissue with increased extracellular space. Since fibrotic atrial tissue is composed of disorganized muscle cells and collagen, and has expanded extracellular space, it is more noticeable with extracellular contrasts [231]. The contrast agent diffuses rapidly out of capillaries after intravenous administration. Since the agent is not able to cross into cells with intact membranes, it accumulates in the extracellular space. This leads to contrast accumulation in the fibrotic areas in patients with atrial fibrosis. Therefore, fibrotic tissue is visualized with higher signal intensity in comparison with healthy myocardium in T1-weighted MRI scans. Image contrast between fibrotic and normal tissues is increased in LGE-MRI using magnetization preparation by inversion or saturation radiofrequency pulses [232].

The DECAAF study [233] was a multicenter study conducted at 15 clinical centers that have adopted the LGE-MRI protocol for left atrial fibrosis into their clinical practice. In this study, subjects assigned for atrial fibrosis imaging underwent 3-dimensional (3D) LGE-MRI along with a contrast-enhanced magnetic resonance angiography and cine imaging in order to define the anatomy of the left atrium and the pulmonary veins [233]. In order to perform the investigation, MRI studies could be performed on 1.5-T and 3-T MRI scanners using either specialized cardiac coils or conventional body and spine phased-array receiver coils. High-resolution LGE images of the left atrium were acquired 15 to 30 min after contrast administration using a 3D inversion-recovery (IR) prepared, respiration navigated, and electrocardiogram (ECG)-triggered gradient-echo pulse sequence with fat saturation. The navigator acceptance window was usually set to ± 3 mm. The data acquisition for LGE sequence is only active if the LA displacement is < 1.5 mm from baseline [233]. In addition, to minimize the effect of LA motion, imaging data were acquired during the diastolic phase of the left atrium with data acquisition limited to 15% of the cardiac cycle. The echo time of the LGE scan was preferably selected to reduce the signal intensity of partial volume fat-tissue voxels and to allow improved delineation of the left atrial wall. The inversion time (TI) value for the LGE-MRI scan was identified using a TI-scout scan. Typical scan time for the LGE-MRI studies take from 8 to 12 min depending on patient rhythm and respiratory pattern [233]. Contraindications for LGE-MRI atrial fibrosis protocol are mainly the same contraindication as for conventional MRI scans: cardiac rhythm devices, severe claustrophobia, and other standard contraindications for MRI at the discretion of the physician, like prosthetic cardiac valves, or paramagnetic material in the brain or in the eyes. Although decreased renal function is not a contraindication, in order to minimize the risk of nephrogenic systemic sclerosis [234], patients with an estimated glomerular filtration rate < 30 ml/min were excluded from fibrosis imaging protocol.

In the DECAAF protocol, MRI data was evaluated and processed by 2 expert operators using Corview image processing and analysis software (Marrek, Salt Lake City, Utah) [233]. The resulting left atrial wall segmentation included the 3D extent of the LA wall and the antral regions of the 4 pulmonary veins. For fibrosis assessment, an algorithm automatically selected intensity thresholds assuming the Gaussian intensity distributions for fibrotic tissue (enhanced voxels) and "normal" myocardium. The threshold was selected based on the estimated mean and standard deviation of "normal" myocardium. The operator validated this threshold by visually inspecting the correspondence between enhanced voxels in LGE-MRI images and algorithm-detected voxels [233]. In the cases of discrepancy, the operator adjusted the threshold to reflect an accurate correspondence. Typical intensity threshold values were in the range of 2 to 4 SDs. The use of the same threshold value for all patients is not feasible because the contrast between normal and fibrotic myocardium in LGE-MRI of the left atrium depends on multiple factors (Table 1)

Searching for atrial substrates using LGE-MRI, the following color coding may be used for 3D visualization of LA fibrosis: healthy tissue is depicted as blue; any other tissue with enhanced LGE is depicted as green and yellow. Moreover, a color lookup-table mask may be applied to better differentiate enhanced from non-enhanced tissue. The processed images are assigned to 1 of the established 4 Utah stages (Figure 3), on the basis of LA wall enhancement as a percentage of the total LA wall volume: stage I, defined as $< 10\%$, stage II ≥ 10 to $< 20\%$, stage III ≥ 20 to $< 30\%$, and stage IV $\geq 30\%$.

Quantification of right atrial fibrosis by LGE-MRI can be performed in a similar fashion [235]. Of note, the correction of the image intensity inhomogeneity and accurate segmentation of the atrial wall are more challenging for the right atrium than for the left atrium because of the proximity to receiver coils and a significant trabeculation of the right atrial free wall.

Table 1. Factors affecting contrast between normal atrium and fibrotic myocardium in LGE-MRI

1. Patient heart rate and rhythm during MRI study.
2. Type and dosage of contrast agent.
3. Time between contrast administration and LGE-MRI scan.
4. Patient-specific contrast clearance rate.
5. Choice of inversion time value for LGE scan.
6. Strength of the main field of MRI scanner.
7. Patient body mass index.
8. Blood hematocrit.
9. Oxygenation level.

With the use of different imaging techniques, catheter ablation of the left atrium is increasingly performed to treat patients with AF. Several approaches to ablation are in use at different centers. Most operators aim to achieve electrical isolation of PV triggers, and some advocate ablation of additional targets [236]. It is very important to study in detail the anatomy of the PV with imaging modalities techniques because of variations in anatomy. Various non-invasive imaging techniques such as MRI and multi-detector computed tomography have shown a variable pulmonary vein anatomy among patients. An example of this variability is the number of PVs: some patients have 5 distinct ostia while others have common trunks. A common left or right pulmonary vein is seen in 25% [236-239] being more frequently on the left than the right PVs. The existence of "extra" PVs, the most common is a separate right middle PV draining the middle lobe of the lung, is another common finding [240] present in up to 26% of patients [241]. The ostial diameter of this right middle PV is smaller than other veins. The classic arrangement of 4 orifices of PV is found in 74%, with 31% of these in the setting of a short vestibule or funnel-like common vein. Five venous orifices were found in 17%, and the remaining 9% had a common vein on the left or right side [242]. In the classic pattern, the right superior PV passes behind the junction between the right atrium and the superior cava vein, whereas the right inferior PV passes behind the inter-cava area. The orifices of the right PVs are directly adjacent to the plane of the atrial septum. Of course, variations in PV anatomy are limitations to successful PV isolation with catheter circumferential AF ablation [242-245]. This is only one reason why innovations in imaging modalities and ablation techniques are emerging.

Late-gadolinium enhancement MRI has been shown to identify areas of fibrosis [246-248] and scarring in the left atrium before and after ablation [248-250]. The predictive value of atrial tissue fibrosis prior to ablation in predicting arrhythmia recurrence following ablation has been demonstrated. The amount of ablation-induced scarring has been suggested to be an important predictor of arrhythmia recurrence [248, 249].

There are different techniques that may be used to obtain images with enhanced LGE-MRI, however, it is good to know that there is certain agreement on the MRI techniques used by different clinical centers. The techniques utilized for the assessment of LA fibrosis and post-ablation scar are similar to those used for the DECAAF study. All groups are using ECG-triggered, respiratory navigated gradient echo pulse sequences with IR preparation and fat saturation. The pulse sequence is acquired 15 to 30 min after administration of 0.1 to 0.2 mmol/kg of gadolinium based contrast agent. Besides Corview, two other tailored software packages are in use to assess atrial fibrosis, Itk-SNAP Version 2.2.0 [251] and QMass MR Software Version 7.2 (Medis Medical Imaging Systems, Leiden, the Netherlands) [252]. The main difference between the centers performing assessment of LA fibrosis is how LGE images are analyzed to quantify LA fibrosis. The majority utilized manual or semi-manual approaches to segment the LA walls from LGE images. In addition, in order to visualize better the atrial endocardial surface, contrast enhanced magnetic resonance angiography acquired at the same cardiac and respiratory phases as 3D LGE-MRI can be used to simplify segmentation of LA endocardial surface. This is an operator-dependent section of images acquired. Therefore, some laboratories quantify LA fibrosis analyzing signal intensity distribution of the segmented LA walls and relying on expert operator decision to select detection thresholds, which typically range from 2 to 4 SDs above the mean for normal myocardium [253-256]. Other centers use the LA blood pool as a reference to identify enhanced LA wall voxels [257-261]. The image intensity ratio method proposed by Khurram et al. [258] normalizes the intensity of the LA wall by the mean value of the blood pool intensity. This approach may reduce intra-operator and inter-operator variability in quantification of LA fibrosis. Fukumoto K et al. [259] utilized an image intensity ratio > 0.97 to identify pre-existing LGE, and an image intensity ratio > 1.61 to identify preexisting dense LGE, respectively. On the other hand, Benito EM et al. [262] has utilized an image intensity ratio < 1.2 to identify healthy atrial myocardium, an image intensity ratio between 1.2 and 1.32 for interstitial fibrosis, and an image intensity ratio > 1.32 for dense scarring. The discrepancy in image intensity ratio thresholds between different centers may be attributed to the fact that these laboratories have used MRI scanners with different field strengths, different contrast agents, and different time intervals between contrast administration and LGE-MRI acquired images. These and several other factors can change the ratio of image intensities of myocardium and blood pool. Furthermore, this ratio is dependent on the inversion time value, the heart rate and rhythm during MRI acquisition, a patient-specific contrast clearance rate, the BMI, blood hematocrit, and oxygenation level.

Despite of these inconveniences, the inter-observer variability demonstrated a high reproducibility. The inter-observer variability of LA fibrosis assessment has been studied and well-reported by some centers. The CARMA study researchers have reported inter-observer correlation coefficients in the range of 0.79 to 0.97, which demonstrate high reproducibility with respect to segmentation of LA wall and fibrosis quantification [253-256]. Other experienced centers reported a correlation coefficient of 0.93 with respect to quantification of LGE, with a reported inter-observer agreement of 0.96 [255]. Such high correlation coefficients for observer variability are a reflection of experience in acquisition of good quality LGE-MRI scans, accurate segmentation of LA wall, and reproducible fibrosis quantification in high-volume centers.

Due to several factors influencing changes in the ratio of image intensities of atrial myocardium, there are several challenges in atrial fibrosis imaging that are of major concern. Right atrial walls measuring 2 to 4 mm are up to 3-fold thinner than ventricular walls (Figure 6) [263]. Considering a spatial resolution of 1.2 to 1.5 mm of LGE-MRI scans, the partial volume effect from surrounding tissue bears the risk of wrongly characterizing adjacent tissue as LA wall (Figure 7) [264]. In order to improve spatial resolution, a prolonged acquisition time may be used. Although, longer acquisition times may result in reduced contrast between fibrotic and normal tissue because T1 relaxation time of tissue can change significantly due to contrast clearance [265]. Therefore, scanners with higher field strength might achieve better spatial resolution. Second, due to the limited spatial resolution of LGE-MRI scans, it remains a challenge to differentiate between transmural and partial thickness of left atrial fibrosis. In addition, data acquisition for LGE-MRI of atrial walls cannot be performed within a single heart cycle. Hence, the data acquisition process has to be ECG-triggered and limited to less than 20% of the RR intervals with adjustment of the acquisition window duration and position depending on the heart rate and rhythm. The QRS complex has to be accurately detected by the scanner to ensure that data are acquired at the same time of cardiac cycle for adequate gating [266]. Data acquisition is performed in atrial diastole to minimize motion artifacts and extend data acquisition duration.

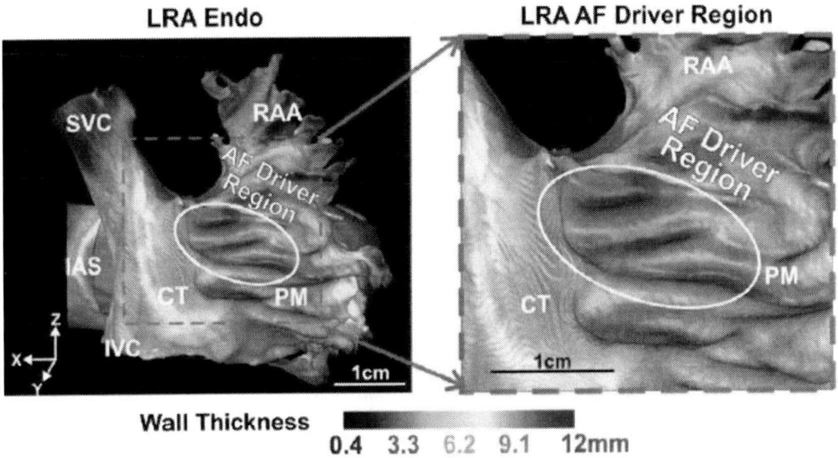

Figure 6. Three-dimensional (3D) atrial wall thickness variation across the whole human atria. In the left, 3D wall thickness of the LRA is superimposed on the atrial endocardium and displayed from the right lateral view. In the right, enhanced view of the AF driver region in the LRA. The white ovals indicate the locations of AF driver regions defined by optical mapping. AF indicates atrial fibrillation. CT: crista terminalis. Endo: endocardium. IAS: interatrial septum. IVC/SVC: inferior/superior vena cava. RA: right atrium. LAA/RAA: left/right atrial appendage. LRA: lateral right atrium. PMs, pectinate muscles. Reprinted with permission from Zhao J, Hansen BJ, Wang Y, Csepe TA, Sul LV, Tang A, et al. Three-dimensional Integrated Functional, Structural, and Computational Mapping to Define the Structural "Fingerprints" of Heart-Specific Atrial Fibrillation Drivers in Human Heart *Ex Vivo*. J Am Heart Assoc. 2017; 6: e005922. DOI: 10.1161/JAHA.117.005922.

In contrast to patients in sinus rhythm with stable RR intervals, imaging of the left atrium in atrial fibrillation or frequent premature beats remains a challenge. For such patients, data acquisition should be performed early after the R-wave, and the duration of the data acquisition window should be shortened to 10% or 12% of the average RR interval. On the other hand, since conventional breath-hold imaging with long breath-holds is often challenging for patients with cardiopulmonary disease, a respiratory gating algorithm is applied in order to minimize respiratory motion artifacts [267].

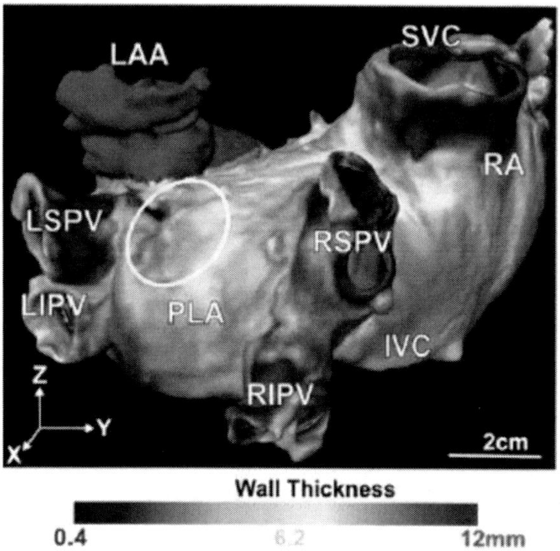

Figure 7. Structural fingerprints in the superior PLA driver region. Three-dimensional (3D) bi-atrial wall thickness of the human atria is superimposed on the atrial epicardium and displayed at the posterior roof view. The white ovals indicate the location of the superior PLA driver region suggested by optical mapping. IVC/SVC: inferior/superior vena cava. RA: right atrium. LAA: left atrial appendage. LSPV/LIPV/RSPV/RIPV: left superior/left inferior/right superior/right inferior pulmonary vein. PLA: posterior left atrium. Reprinted with permission from Zhao J, Hansen BJ, Wang Y, Csepe TA, Sul LV, Tang A, et al. Three-dimensional Integrated Functional, Structural, and Computational Mapping to Define the Structural "Fingerprints" of Heart-Specific Atrial Fibrillation Drivers in Human Heart *Ex Vivo*. J Am Heart Assoc. 2017; 6: e005922. DOI: 10.1161/JAHA.117.005922.

Despite these mentioned issues, pooled data from the CARMA center and from Cochet et al. [255] reveal that appropriate images for quantification of left atrial fibrosis can be obtained in 83% to 100% of LGE-MRIs [255-257]. In a retrospective analysis of DECAAF data, errors of the attending technologist were identified as the primary source [62%] of poor quality scans (Table 2).

It was also demonstrated that 31% of the poor quality scans were patient-related, and 7% were the result of hardware issues. With respect to patient-related issues, arrhythmia and irregular respiratory patterns were causative for poor image quality at the same 40% incidence. Both overall image quality and fibrosis/scar visibility of LGE-MRI of the left atrium depend on the heart rate and regularity of heart rhythm [268]. Vijayakumar S et al. [269] have shown a significantly lower scar visibility in patients with a heart rate greater than 100 beats per min.

Table 2. Causes of poor quality image scans

A. Mistakes of the attending technologist.
1. Wrong inversion time-scout scan value.
2. Wrong phase-encoding direction.
3. Errors in navigator prescription.
4. Partial coverage of the left atrium.
B. Patient-related poor quality scans.
1. Irregular cardiac arrhythmias.
2. Tachycardias.
3. Irregular respiratory patterns.
C. Hardware-related poor quality scans.
1. Ghosting artifacts.
2. LA wall blurring resulting of hardware issues.
3. Scans acquired by old generations of 1.5-T scanners.

Higuchi K, et al. [270] recently studied the spatial distribution of LGE-MRI of the left atrium in patients with AF. They performed LGE-MRI scans to 160 patients with AF with a mean age 66 ± 11 years before AF ablation. In order to know the spatial distribution of LGE, the extent of LGE in 6 LA sub-regions was examined. Overall LGE distribution was also summarized as a spatial frequency histogram using an atlas of LA shape. Their data were also compared between paroxysmal AF (87 patients) and persistent AF (73 patients). The authors found that LGE coverage (%) in each sub-region was as follows: 41.8 ± 18.9% in the left pulmonary vein (PV) antrum, 27.1 ± 16.7% in the left lateral wall, 25.8 ± 15.3% in the posterior wall, 19.7 ± 15.3% in the anterior wall, 17.1 ± 15.0% in the right PV antrum, and 12.0 ± 13.2% in the septum wall. LGE was heterogeneously distributed in the LA and was found with the highest frequency in the posterior wall near the inferior left PV antrum by the LGE histogram. A comparison of paroxysmal AF with persistent AF suggests that LGE was more expected in persistent

AF compared with paroxysmal AF, particularly with a spread on the posterior and the anterior wall. Therefore, they concluded that LGE in the LA was heterogeneously distributed. LGE was highly distributed in the inferior left PV antrum near the posterior wall side, and spread on the posterior and anterior wall with AF progression [270].

Platonov PG, et al. [271], observed that the LA posterior wall at the inferior PV level was the only time-dependent area of significant fibrosis in a histological study of autopsied human hearts. Tanaka K, et al. [272] found that LA fibrosis in the posterior wall and the PV antrum played a significant role in maintaining AF in an experimental study using a sheep AF model with heart failure [272]. Using patients with chronic AF who underwent mitral valve surgery and autopsied control, Corradi D, et al. [273] also demonstrated that fibrosis occurs more in the LA posterior wall than in the left atrial appendage. Higuchi K, et al. [270] supposed that the heterogeneous LGE distribution in their study patients in particular LA regions is derived from the external structures around the LA. More LA remodeling could occur due to a mechanical pressure or a friction with the aorta, esophagus, and vertebral body [274]. The proximity of the LA posterior wall and the descending aorta can be recognized at the left inferior PV ostium level where mechanical friction may occur [275]. The vertebral body and ascending aorta attach more on the dilated LA wall as AF progress, and increase remodeling on the attached area, namely, posterior and anterior LA wall. That can be an explanation why LGE spreads on the posterior wall and occurs on the anterior wall when progressing from paroxysmal AF to persistent AF.

Lachman N, et al. [276] stated that the pressure stress other than the mechanical friction to the LA wall also varies due to different pericardial structures, resulting in heterogeneity of LGE. In a study by Hunter et al. [277], 3D computed tomography scans were used to estimate the wall pressure stress in patients with persistent AF. Wall stress was particularly common around left PV ostia and the left atrial appendage ridge. Nakahara S, et al. [278] demonstrated that areas of pivot activation during AF which were cores of localized activation in AF were found at the anterior wall, left

PV antrum, and posterior wall where external structures such as the aorta and the vertebral body attached.

When Higuchi K, et al. [270] compared LGE distribution in patients with paroxysmal AF and persistent AF, no difference was seen on the left PV antrum and the left lateral wall. Although a significantly greater LGE distribution was observed in patients with persistent AF in other areas, especially on the posterior wall and the anterior wall. This result suggests that LGE was common on the left PV antrum or the left lateral wall. This was observed even in patients with paroxysmal AF with rather healthy LA myocardium, and then occurs in other areas of the atrial walls as disease progresses to persistent AF [270].

The STAR AF II trial, a large, multicenter, randomized trial that performed substrate and trigger ablation for AF reduction showed that empiric linear ablation or complex fractionated electrogram ablation did not have a benefit compared with simple PV isolation in patients with persistent AF [279]. The importance of LGE of the left atrium for AF recurrence prediction after ablation was already reported several years ago [280-283]. More recent studies also showed the importance of low voltage zone in AF ablation. By additional modification of the zones with low voltage electrograms in the left atrium, the rate of AF recurrence was decreased only by PV isolation [284-287]. Therefore, knowing the sites of low voltage zone appearance is now an increasing concern. Evaluating the site-specific LGE appearance before AF ablation might be useful, in additional modification at remodeled site of the left atrium together with PV isolation.

About 15 years ago, noninvasive electrocardiographic imaging mapping has been introduced for real-time and whole-heart mapping of cardiac electrical activity [288]. The technique was validated versus high-density contact mapping in animals [289, 290]. It has also been applied in humans to study ventricular and atrial arrhythmias [291-293], and conduction disturbances in heart failure [294]. In patients with persistent AF, regions harboring reentrant activity can be identified by phase map calculation from either contact data acquired with bi-atrial basket catheters [295], or noncontact data acquired by electrocardiographic imaging mapping [292]. Using these methods, clinical reports have demonstrated the benefit of a tailored ablation approach targeting patient-specific re-entrant drivers [295, 296]. Conversely, interstitial fibrosis is consistently present in patients with AF [297, 298]. Experimental data have shown that re-entry can be induced and maintained by both electrophysiological and structural remodeling and that fibrosis plays a major role in the mechanisms of fibrillation organization [299-302]. Developments in cardiac MRI techniques now enable the acquisition of LGE images with sufficient spatial resolution to study the atrial wall [303]. Because gadolinium-based contrast agents have an interstitial distribution, areas of LGE in the atrium represent areas where interstitial fibrosis is the most pronounced, as corroborated by histological studies [304]. In this context, Cochet H, et al. [305] assessed the relationship between fibrosis and re-entrant activity in 41 patients with persistent AF (age 56 ± 12 years). They performed high-resolution electrocardiographic imaging (ECGI) during AF by using a 252-chest electrode array. Phase mapping was applied to locate re-entrant activity. Sites of high re-entrant activity were defined as re-entrant regions. LGE-MRI was performed at 1.25 x 1.25 x 2.5 mm resolution to characterize atrial fibrosis and measure atrial volumes. The relationship between LGE burden and the number of re-entrant regions was analyzed. Local LGE density was computed and characterized at re-entrant sites. All their patients underwent catheter ablation targeting re-entrant regions, the procedural endpoint being AF termination. Clinical, cardiac LGE-MRI, and ECGI predictors of acute procedural success were analyzed. They found that left atrial LGE burden was 22.1 ± 5.9% of the wall, and left atrial volume was 74 ± 21 ml/m2. The number of re-entrant regions was 4.3 ± 1.7 per patient. Left atrial LGE imaging was significantly associated with the number of re-entrant regions ($R = 0.52$; $p = 0.001$), with left atrial volume ($R = 0.62$; $p < 0.0001$), and with AF duration ($R = 0.54$; $p = 0.0007$). Regional analysis demonstrated a clustering of re-entrant activity at LGE borders. Areas with high re-entrant activity showed higher local LGE density as compared with the remaining atrial areas ($p < 0.0001$). In addition, failure to achieve AF termination during catheter ablation was associated with higher left atrial LGE-MRI burden ($p < 0.001$), higher number of re-entrant regions ($p < 0.001$), and longer AF duration ($p = 0.008$). Therefore, the authors concluded that the number of re-entrant regions during AF relates to the extent of LGE on cardiac MRI, with the location of these regions clustering to LGE areas. These characteristics affect procedural outcomes of ablation [305].

These findings are consistent with previous studies [303], and it supports the use of LGE-MRI prior to AF ablation to assess atrial fibrosis and remodeling. Although, Cochet H, et al. [305] also quantified LGE-MRI on the right atrium, the relationships with clinical characteristics were weaker than in the left atrium. This finding suggested that LGE-MRI assessment of fibrosis is less robust on the right atrium than on the left atrium. However, this could also reflect a distinct mechanism of re-entry because of anatomical, structural or functional differences between the left and right atrium [306].

Jadidi AS, et al. [307] demonstrated an inverse relationship between the extent of LGE-MRI and the AF cycle length as measured in the left atrial appendage in a clinical study in patients with persistent AF. Thus, a growing body of evidence suggests that fibrosis burden is related to the global complexity of AF mechanisms. In a recent study in patients with persistent AF, Chrispin J, et al. [308] reported a lack of regional association between atrial LGE and rotors identified using the focal impulse and rotor mapping technology. However, a growing body of evidence supports the role of fibrosis in anchoring re-entry during AF. These findings come from a series of experimental and modeling studies [300-302, 309-311], as well as, from a prior clinical study reporting a clustering of complex fractionated atrial electrograms around atrial fibrotic areas as assessed with LGE-MRI [307].

In an interesting prospective case-control study, Bouazizi K, et al. [198] hypothesized that MRI, when used in an optimal *ex vivo* setting allowing high spatial resolution without motion artifacts, can help characterizing the complex 3D left atrial wall composition in human myocardial samples, as compared to histology. 3D MRI acquisitions including saturation-recovery T1 mapping and 4.0 T DIXON imaging was performed on 9 human left atrial samples collected from patients who underwent cardiac surgery. Histological quantification of fibrosis and fat was obtained. MRI T1 maps were clustered based on a Gaussian Mixture Model allowing quantification of total, interstitial and fatty fibrosis components. Fat maps were computed from DIXON images and fat fractions were calculated. MRI measurements were performed on the same location and plane as the histological analysis and on the entire 3D sample volume. The authors found high correlations and levels of agreement between MRI and histology for total (r = 0.93), interstitial (r = 0.93) and fatty fibrosis (r = 0.98) and fat (r = 0.96) (Figure 8). Native T1 correlated with the amount of fibrosis from MRI and histology. The 3D MRI total, interstitial and fatty fibrosis ranges were between 6% and 23%, 4% and 17.3%; and 1.4% and 19.7% respectively. Therefore, they concluded that high field *ex vivo* MRI was able to quantify different left atrial myocardial components with high agreement in 2D with histology and moreover to provide 3D quantification of such components whereas *in vivo* application remains a challenge. Nevertheless, Bouazizi K, et al. [198] investigating the ability of MRI to quantify atrial fibrosis subtypes, namely, total, interstitial and fatty demonstrated a high correlation (r = 0.93, P = 0.0007) between MRI and histology in terms of total fibrosis fraction. The Bland-Altman analysis showed good agreement between the two measurements as revealed by a mean difference of - 0.46% and 95% limits of agreement from - 3.32% to 2.4%. Interstitial fibrosis fraction measured from MRI was also highly correlated to histology (r = 0.93, P = 0.0007) and Bland-Altman analysis revealed excellent agreement as shown by a mean difference of 0.24% and 95% limits of agreement from - 1.75% to 2.23%. Fatty fibrosis fraction from MRI was also highly correlated to histology (r = 0.98, P < 0.0001) and Bland-Altman analysis revealed very good agreement as shown by a mean difference of - 0.59% and 95% limits of agreement from - 4.94% to 3.74%. The fibrosis fraction computed in the whole 3D volume from MRI ranged between 6% and 23% for total fibrosis, between 4% and 17.3% for interstitial fibrosis, between 1.4% and 19.7% for fatty fibrosis fractions. Correlations between 3D and 2D measurements were r = 0.76 (P = 0.02) for total fibrosis fraction, r = 0.81 (P = 0.01) for interstitial fibrosis fraction and r = 0.60 (P = 0.09) for fatty fibrosis fraction. Mean native T1 values measured in all samples ranged between 923 and 1285 ms (1154 ± 124 ms). In all samples, fibrotic areas presented higher native T1 values (1131 ± 89 ms) than non-fibrotic myocardium (T1 values = 962 ± 21 ms). Native mean T1 values presented a significant and positive correlation with interstitial MRI fibrosis fraction (r = 0.41, P = 0.01) and trends for a positive correlation but not significant with total (r = 0.41, P = 0.26) MRI fibrosis fraction (r = 0.78, P = 0.01) and a negative correlation with fatty fibrosis (r = - 0.52, P = 0.16) and fat MRI fraction (r = - 0.68, P = 0.05). The authors also found that native mean T1 values presented a significant and positive correlation with interstitial histological fibrosis fraction (r = 0.71, P = 0.03) but not with total histological fibrosis (r = 0.28, P = 0.46) and a negative trend of correlation with fatty fibrosis (r = - 0.53, P = 0.14) and fat histological fraction (r = -0.60, P = 0.09). Overall, the higher correlation coefficient was found between native T1 and interstitial fibrosis fraction from MRI without reaching statistical significance (P = 0.07). These are interesting results since they revealed that when MRI T1 mapping and fat imaging are used in the optimal *ex vivo* settings, with no motion or flow artifacts, high spatial resolution and free of blood signal, they are able to accurately characterize different myocardial components at the tissue level including total fibrosis, interstitial fibrosis, adipose tissue and fibrotic fat in the human left atrial wall (Figure 8). However, it is not currently possible to apply the *ex vivo* T1 mapping sequence used here *in vivo* in a moving heart with a sufficient spatial resolution to reliably study the thin left atrial wall. Further studies should be performed to overcome the challenging technical issues which will allow translation of the observed data to a moving heart.

In the case of hardware issues, the type of scanner has a major impact on the quality of LGE-MRI imaging of the left atrium. The image quality on 1.5- and 3-T scanners revealed poor image quality in 20% of scans acquired by old generations of 1.5-T scanners. The 3-T or modern 1.5-T scanners with specialized cardiac coils are preferable for LGE-MRI of left atrial images. The DECAAF study [233] clearly showed a significant learning curve with the number of patients assessed. Progress in imaging techniques and scanner hardware, as well as better training of MRI technologists, may further improve image quality of LGE-MRI of the left atrium. Additional research studies are needed to analyze further how re-entries anchor to specific atrial substrate areas and particularly to discriminate between structural and functional re-entry mechanisms. Assessment of structural remodeling and atrial arrhythmia mechanisms during AF is feasible by combining LGE-MRI with ECGI data. This multimodal noninvasive approach may be of value to personalize biophysical models, with major potential applications for diagnosis, prognosis, and therapy.

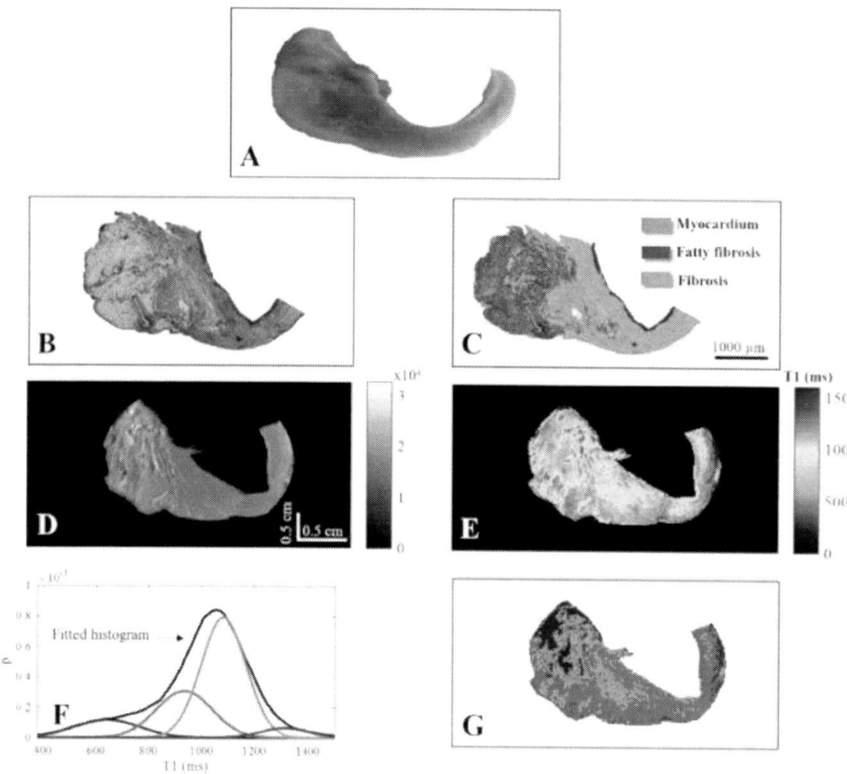

Figure 8. Representative left atrial sample (histology and MRI). (A) Representative left atrial sample (macroscopy), (B) photomicrograph of the Picro-Sirius stained section showing adipose tissue, fibrotic remodeling and myocardium and (C) semi-automated quantitative analysis identifying fibrosis, fibrotic changes in adipose tissue, and myocytes; 10X magnification, scale bar 1000 µm. (D) RARE image of the same sample acquired at TE/TR = 11.4 ms/6.5 s, FOV = 3.84 cmx1.92 cm, matrix = 192x96, (E) T1 map, (F) T1 histogram with 4 Gaussian distributions and the corresponding clustering map in (G). Reprinted with permission from Bouazizi K, Rahhal A, Kusmia S, Evin M, Defrance C, Cluzel P, et al. (2018) Differentiation and quantification of fibrosis, fat and fatty fibrosis in human left atrial myocardium using *ex vivo* MRI. PLoS ONE 2018; 13(10): e0205104. https://doi.org/10.1371/journal.pone.0205104.

USE OF 3D ELECTROANATOMIC MAPPING FOR IMAGING OF ATRIAL FIBROSIS

3D electroanatomic mapping (3D EAM) has been successfully used for several years in clinical electrophysiological studies for atrial fibrosis and atrial substrate description [312-322]. Kottkamp H, et al. [318] described their AF ablation procedure stating that 3D EAM was performed during sinus rhythm. Even in patients with persistent AF where electrical cardioversion cannot restore a stable sinus rhythm before pulmonary vein (PV) isolation, the procedure started first with PV isolation then followed by electrical cardioversion to restore sinus rhythm. This approach allowed mapping during normal sinus rhythm in almost all patients. Then, they created a left atrial shell with point-by-point acquisition using the ablation catheter and a 3-dimensional mapping system (Carto-3, Biosense Webster, Diamond Bar, California). A computer tomography 3D reconstruction of the left atrium was merged with the 3D EA voltage mapping shell. The mapping points were homogenously distributed within the left atrium with denser sampling at the posterior/inferior/superior and anterior/septal walls, and somewhat less dense sampling at the mitral isthmus region and within the left atrial appendage. Adequate catheter-tissue contact was indicated by stable contact force sensing (5 to 10 g), and only points during stable sinus rhythm were acquired. The Carto system annotated peak-to-peak electrogram amplitudes for automatic measurement of bipolar electrogram amplitude. Kottkamp H, et al. [318] stated that all acquired mapping points were manually reviewed for correctness of automatic measurement. For color coding of 3D EA voltage mapping, voltages <0.5 mV were colored red, and voltages > 1.5 mV were colored purple. The procedural technique for 3D EAM is still developing and future advances are awaited. The methodology to describe the fibrotic substrate using 3D EA voltage mapping during sinus rhythm is under investigation and several limitations remain at this point in time. Several variables still influence and act as limiting factors. The measured voltage depends on the cardiac rhythm, the contact of the electrode to the tissue, the thickness of the atrial myocardium, the electrode size and spacing, the wave front direction, and other variables [313, 318].

In an effort for defining scars and their role in AF ablation, Verma A, et al. [319] described in patients who underwent PV antrum isolation, that pre-existent left atrial "scarring" in their AF ablation patients was an independent predictor of procedural failure. Low voltage for "abnormal" areas was defined as an amplitude $\leq$ 0.5 mV, and "scar" $\leq$ 0.05 mV indistinguishable from noise. Kapa S, et al. [320] recently described in their AF patients undergoing catheter ablation that contact 3D EAM derived voltage criteria was good enough for characterizing left atrial "scar". In their study, a voltage range of 0.2 to 0.45 mV was found to delineate "scar." Other researchers [321] utilized 0.2 to 0.5 mV as "diseased" atria, and > 0.5 mV as "healthy" atria. In addition, others used values of 0.5 to 1.5 mV to represent an "intermediate" zone that does not mean "severe" fibrosis but also not "normal" atrial myocardium.

It is interesting to note, that the fragmented electrogram appearance of voltages in the range of 0.5 and 1.5 mV argue toward mild/moderate fibrosis. In some cases, these fragmented electrograms can even be found at voltages of 1.5 to 2.5 mV [313]. The evidence tells that there are different grades in atrial fibrosis and these differences can be described by 3D EA voltage mapping. Kottkamp H, et al. [318] proposed the terms "severe fibrosis" for sites with voltages < 0.5 mV, an intermediate zone with "mild/moderate fibrosis" for sites with voltages of 0.5 to 1.5 mV, and "less affected or normal" for sites with voltages > 1.5 mV. An atrial "scar" was defined only for sites with no discrete electrograms and no local capture during pacing. There is an exception in the anterior sites with overlying epicardial Bachmann bundle, where atrial muscle fibers within severe fibrosis can be present at sites with voltages about or even below 0.05 mV. A similar methodology was described by Yang G, et al. [322] stating a definition of severely affected areas with voltages < 0.4 mV and a "transitional" zone of 0.4 to 1.3 mV. However, the necessary overall spatial mapping resolution for adequately describing the fibrotic substrate is unclear. There are different and several conceptions on the number of atrial mapping points. Some used a mean of 140 left atrial mapping points [320], others used 54 to 158 (mean: 115) points [321], and 100 to 130 mapping points [313], or even 140 to 200 points in some patients [317]. With the use of multipolar electrode catheters with constant automatic acquisition of mapping points one can obtain a higher number of mapping points (e.g., > 500 or even > 1,000 points), with the limitation of acceptance of mapping points without contact (e.g., within 5 mm of the atrial surface) and with limited/no option for verification of annotation.

The amplitude of atrial electrograms obtained by 3D EA voltage mapping may also vary depending on several variables. Indeed, bipolar as well as unipolar electrogram amplitudes are influenced by electrode size, by inter-electrode spacing, by contact versus noncontact sites, and by the activation wave front direction in relation to the orientation of the mapping catheter. Anter E, et al. [323] compared atrial mapping with a 3.5-mm electrode tip catheter with a 1-mm multi-electrode mapping catheter (Pentaray, Biosense Webster). In control patients, normal bipolar voltage amplitudes were similar between 3.5-mm and 1.0-mm electrode catheters. In patients with scar-related atrial arrhythmias, the total area of bipolar voltage < 0.50 mV was smaller with the 1-mm electrode catheter (14.7 vs. 20.4 cm2), and the mean bipolar voltage amplitude in this area was higher (0.28 vs. 0.17 mV) [323].

On the other hand, atrial electrograms obtained during AF by 3D EA voltage mapping show a considerable temporal variability of electrogram amplitude and morphology. Yagishita A, et al. [324] recently compared left atrial electrograms voltage during sinus rhythm and during AF in the same patient. Mapping points were manually selected aiming to represent approximate median peak-to-peak bipolar voltage amplitude. All atrial electrograms obtained during 10 consecutive QRS complexes were quantitatively measured. These investigators found a significantly higher left atrial bipolar voltage in sinus rhythm compared with AF but a linear voltage correlation between sinus rhythm and AF [324]. Potentially, voltage mapping findings could then be combined with activation mapping data during ongoing AF. Furthermore, in their control group, 95% of voltage distribution outside the PV were > 1.46 mV [324].

3D EA voltage mapping allowed identification of areas with atrial fibrosis that can later on be targeted for AF ablation. The individual regional localization of areas with severe fibrosis allows the application of the circumferential isolation of substantially affected fibrotic areas (< 0.5 mV) [313, 318]. These ablation lines are, in general, connected to the PV isolation lines to prevent the production of small channels and their potential pro-arrhythmic effect. This strategy was originally tested and validated in redo patients with paroxysmal AF who presented with AF recurrences despite durable PV isolation by Kottkamp H, et al. [313]. In 9 of 10 patients, regional areas of severe fibrosis (< 0.5 mV) could be identified. In 1 of 10 patients, a confluent large area of moderately reduced voltage (0.5 to 2.5 mV) was revealed at the anteroseptal LA wall. In this area with moderately reduced voltage, fragmented bipolar electrograms were taken as an additional surrogate for fibrosis. Complete isolation was confirmed with a multipolar circular mapping catheter. During a mean follow-up of 20 months, 9 of 10 patients remained in sinus rhythm after atrial fibrosis ablation [313]. These authors then extended this strategy to first procedures in patients with non-paroxysmal AF [318]. In 13 of 31 patients (42%), no or very limited low-voltage areas were found. In these 13 cases, only PV isolation was performed. During a mean follow-up of 16 ± 7 months, 9 of 13 patients (69%) stayed in stable sinus rhythm after a single procedure, and 11 of 13 patients (85%) were in sinus rhythm after multiple procedures (1.15 per patient). In 18 of 31 patients (58%), areas of severe fibrosis were recorded. During a follow-up of 12 ± 5 months, 14 of 18 patients (78%) stayed in stable sinus rhythm after a single procedure and 15 of 18 patients (83%) were in sinus rhythm after 1.1 procedures per patient. With respect to the overall non-paroxysmal AF group, 23 of 31 patients (74%) were free from AF or atrial tachycardia after a single procedure during a follow-up of 14 ± 6 months and 26 of 31 patients (84%) after 1.13 procedures per patient.

Considering these results, it is well appreciated that in a subgroup of patients with persistent AF, only PV isolation is needed. However, no clear selection criteria for that conservative approach had been elaborated beyond achievability of sinus rhythm after PV isolation with electrical cardioversion. AF ablation was restricted to only PV isolation in non-paroxysmal AF patients with no or very limited fibrosis [313, 318]. Despite this limited ablation approach, freedom of AF/atrial tachycardia reached 85% with only 1.15 procedures per patient. This provides a new selection criterion for PV isolation-only ablation in non-paroxysmal AF patients [313, 318]. On the contrary, in patients with extensive fibrosis as indicated by 3D EA voltage mapping, it is discouraged to perform even a second ablation procedure. This is because the likelihood of achieving stable sinus rhythm is very low. This fact is in accordance to other reports using 3D EA voltage mapping, as well as, LGE-MRI showing that extensive left atrial fibrosis is an important predictor of AF ablation failure and recurrence [319, 325].

On the other hand, the arrhythmogenic role of confluent areas of mild fibrosis needs further investigation. In general, it is not the presence of fibrosis per se, but the interplay between the myocardial fibers and the fibrosis fibers on a microscopic scale that permits or not the myocardial fibers to perpetuate the complex activation pattern resulting in AF. In contrast, replacement fibrosis without interconnecting muscle fibers does not necessarily need to be arrhythmogenic. However, the critical areas of mappable atrial tachycardia after PV isolation in AF patients are typically located in areas of severe fibrosis (< 0.5 mV) [313, 318]. Schreiber D, et al. [314] analyzed fibrosis distribution and extent, clinical characteristics, and their impact on rhythm outcome in 141 patients. Forty-nine AF patients without atrial fibrosis were treated with PV isolation only, and 92 patients with mild to moderate atrial fibrosis were treated with PV isolation plus atrial fibrosis ablation. Single and multiple procedure (1.1 per patient) success rates at 12 months were almost identical in these two groups nearly 90%, whereas in patients with extensive fibrosis, it was only 41% and 61% (with 1.2 per patient). However, the weaker outcome in this subgroup was mainly driven by patients with the most severe atrial fibrosis showing only a success rate of 20% [314]. In multivariate models, fibrosis measures were significantly associated with single and multiple procedure outcomes, whereas clinical characteristics of the patients as age, hypertension, and diabetes were not correlated with the size of severe fibrosis areas. The importance of mild fibrosis was recently addressed in a study by Yagishita A, et al. [325], in which mildly affected areas defined as <1.1 mV were an independent predictor for arrhythmia recurrence in AF patients without severe fibrosis < 0.5 mV undergoing PV isolation alone.

Rolf S, et al. [321] also described a tailored substrate modification based on voltage criteria. They used a combination of ablation strategies including linear lines through low-voltage areas as well as encircling of low-voltage areas and also "homogenization," and they used several endpoints including a significant reduction in local electrograms, defractionation, and loss of capture [321]. Reduction in electrogram amplitude may not be a typical finding of isolation. After isolation of posterior, superior, or inferior areas, clear isoelectric lines with no potentials are typically observed after complete isolation. However, in anteroseptal ablation, reduction in amplitude is a typical sign of incomplete isolation with activation of this area through a remaining input of Bachmann bundle [326]. The placement of a linear line through a fibrotic area could ablate a stable arrhythmia. However, preliminary mapping from "AF rotors" have shown a meandering spatial behavior in areas of substantial size. Hence, the "AF rotor" might sustain above or below a linear ablation line. After a long-term median follow-up of 3.1 years, Yagishita A, et al. [327] recently described that 144 of 201 patients (74%) were free from recurrence after multiple procedures including substrate modification in patients with low voltage areas < 0.5mV. In their study, voltage mapping was performed during ongoing AF. Already some years ago, empirical isolation of the posterior wall at the level of the PV without prior 3D EA voltage mapping was introduced [328].

Some researchers have tried to use an interesting approach of homogenizing areas of substantial fibrosis with the intention to achieve atrial electrograms of less than 0.1 mV. Yang G, et al. [322] described a substrate modification approach in patients with non-paroxysmal AF with "homogenization" of areas with low voltage. They tried to ablate all detectable electrograms within the target areas to achieve bipolar electrograms of < 0.1 mV, short linear lesions were placed to ablate potential conduction channels. Voltages of up to 0.5 mV are generated after complete isolation by the adjacent epicardial Bachmann bundle, and these potentials need to be differentiated from left atrial myocardium to prevent unnecessary additional radiofrequency energy applications. A similar approach of homogenizing areas of substantial fibrosis was recently described by Yamaguchi et al. [329]. Freedom from AF was much lower in their study in persistent AF patients with areas of substantial fibrosis who only underwent PV isolation compared with the group undergoing additional substrate modification (38% vs. 72%) [329]. When comparing the approach of homogenization with the circumferential isolation approach in areas of substantial fibrosis measuring 20 cm^2 or even more, the circumferential substrate fibrosis ablation approach might be the more specific strategy with less burning and a clearer endpoint.

In another interesting and recent study, Jadidi AS, et al. [330] combined voltage mapping criteria during ongoing AF (< 0.5 mV) with regional activation criteria in patients with persistent AF. Specifically, focal ablation was done at low-voltage sites associated with electric activity lasting > 70% of AF cycle length on a single electrode (fractionated activity) or multiple electrodes around the circumferential mapping catheter (rotational activity) or discrete rapid local activity with the procedural endpoint of AF termination [330]. The authors stated that arrhythmia freedom was higher in this substrate modification approach group compared with a matched control group of PV isolation only. Interestingly, AF-termination sites co-localized within low-voltage areas in 80% and at border zones in 20% [330]. Seven years ago, in the CONFIRM Trial, the hypothesis was tested that human AF is functionally maintained by localized rotors whose specific elimination might improve outcome after ablation [331]. Indeed, the approach of focal impulse and rotor modulation seems to have better results. Furthermore, images of the biatrial geometry were described by Haissaguerre M, et al. [332] using an array of 252 body surface electrodes plus thoracic computed tomography. These authors utilized a specific signal-analysis process to identify drivers in distinct categories of persistent AF. Using this technology, persistent AF in early months was described to be maintained predominantly by drivers that were found to be clustered in a few regions with most of them being unstable re-entries [332, 333].

Left atrial low voltage substrate potentially slows intra-atrial conduction, which might identify patients at risk for arrhythmia recurrence following pulmonary vein isolation. Up to 50% of the patients with persistent AF have arrhythmia recurrence following pulmonary vein isolation, mostly due to arrhythmogenic left atrial low voltage substrate. In this context, recently Jadidi AS, et al. [334] hypothesized that progressive left atrial remodeling in persistent AF with development of left atrial low voltage substrate leads to intra-atrial conduction slowing that should be measurable using intracardiac activation mapping and be reflected by prolonged P wave duration (PWD) on amplified digitized 12-lead electrocardiography (ECG) (Figure 9). If so, marked prolongation of the amplified sinus rhythm P-wave might predict arrhythmia recurrences in patients with persistent AF undergoing pulmonary vein isolation (Figure 10). The authors performed electrocardioversion to sinus rhythm and high-density voltage mapping of the left atrium in 72 patients with persistent AF. Invasively measured left atrial activation time and PWD were quantitatively measured. Digitized 12-lead ECG were compared with the extent of left atrial low voltage substrate (< 0.5 and < 1. 0mV). Freedom from arrhythmia following PVI was evaluated in 143 patients with persistent AF stratified according to amplified PWD before ablation. They observed that left atrial low voltage substrate resulted in regional conduction delay, which increased LA activation time. In Figure 11 is depicted the correlation found for left atrial low voltage and LA activation time. LA PWD strongly correlated with left atrial activation time ($r = 0.96$) and left atrial low voltage substrate ($r = 0.80$). PWD ≥ 150 ms identified advanced left atrial low voltage substrate with 94.3% sensitivity and 91.7% specificity. One-year arrhythmia freedom following pulmonary vein isolation-only was significantly higher in patients with PWD less than 150 ms ($n = 73$) compared to those with prolonged PWD ≥ 150 ms ($n = 70$) (72.0% vs. 40.8%; $p = 0.003$). Total PWD correlated with left atrial low voltage substrate ($r = 0.84$) (Figure 12). Therefore, the authors concluded that advanced arrhythmogenic low voltage substrate is associated with significant intra-atrial conduction delay, which is accurately measurable by prolongation of PWD on amplified 12-lead ECG. PWD ≥150 ms during sinus rhythm measured prior to ablation identifies patients with persistent AF who are at increased risk for arrhythmia recurrence following pulmonary vein isolation [334].

The study of Jadidi AS, et al. [334] demonstrated that significant left atrial low voltage substrate, as correlate of atrial fibrosis structural remodeling, is present in only some patients with persistent AF. Independent

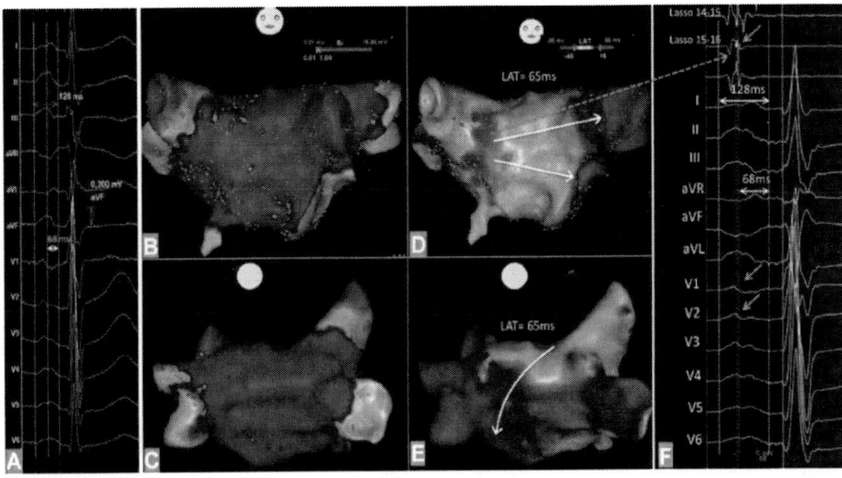

Figure 9. Left Atrial P-Wave Analysis and Corresponding Invasively Measured Left Atrial Activation Time in a Patient Without Relevant Low-Voltage Substrate. (A) Twelve-lead surface electrocardiogram of a representative patient with absence of low voltage. Left atrial P-wave duration (LAP) is measured from the point of highest negative deflection (-dV/dt max) in lead V1 or V2 to the end of the P-wave in any of the leads (here 68 ms). Total P-wave duration is measured from the earliest deflection in any lead to the last point of electric activity in any lead (here 128 ms). Voltage map of the same patient at 1.0-mV cutoff shows no significant low-voltage areas in the anterior (B) and posterior (C) views. (D, E) Activation mapping of this patient demonstrates fast activation that spreads from the septum to the left atrial appendage (65 ms). The earliest activation of the septal left atrium as demonstrated in the activation map corresponds to -dV/dt max in lead V1 or V2. LAT: left atrial activation time. Reprinted with permission from Jadidi A, Müller-Edenborn B, Chen J, Keyl C, Weber R, Allgeier J, et al. The duration of the amplified sinus-P-wave identifies presence of left atrial low voltage substrate and predicts outcome after pulmonary vein isolation in patients with persistent atrial fibrillation. J Am Coll Cardiol EP 2018; 4: 531-543.

of the cutoff value defining low voltage in sinus rhythm (bipolar voltage of < 0.5 mV vs. < 1.0 mV), the extent of left atrial low voltage substrate was highly variable, ranging from less than 5 cm^2 to more than 50 cm^2 of the left atrium. Significant left atrial low voltage substrate is associated with conduction delay within the zone of low voltage substrate. It is important that we can have information about low voltage substrate areas with an easy obtainable single parameter like PWD. In Figure 13 is depicted the extent of left atrial low voltage substrate stratified by P-wave duration. PWD in sinus rhythm greater than 150 ms identifies patients with significant left atrial low voltage substrate with high sensitivity and specificity. Patients with shorter duration P waves of less than 150 ms demonstrated only a mean 1.1 and 4.3 cm^2 of left atrial low voltage substrate at 0.5 and 1.0 mV, respectively. In Figure 14 is depicted arrhythmia freedom following pulmonary vein isolation for persistent atrial fibrillation stratified according to P-wave duration.

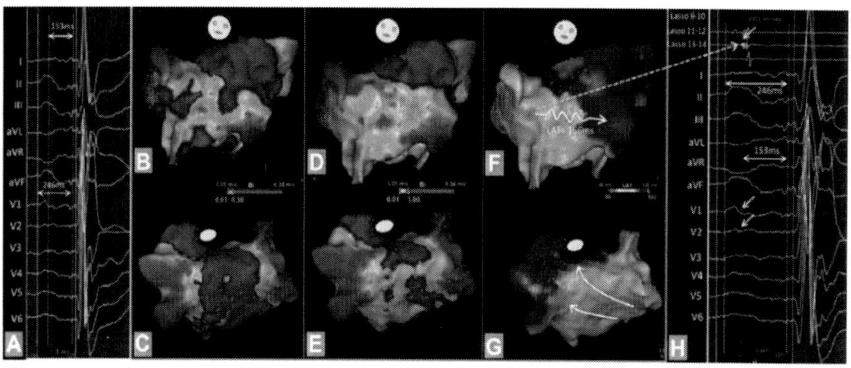

Figure 10. Left Atrial P-Wave Analysis and Corresponding Invasively Measured Left Atrial Activation Time in a Patient With Extensive Low-Voltage Substrate. (A) Twelve-lead surface electrocardiogram of a representative patient with extensive left atrial (LA) low voltage. LA P-wave duration (LAP) is measured from the point of highest negative deflection (-dV/dt max) in lead V1 or V2 to the end of the P-wave in any of the leads (here 153 ms). Voltage mapping shows extensive low voltage of the left atrium both at 0.5-mV (B, C) and 1.0-mV (D, E) cutoffs. LA activation is importantly prolonged (LA activation time [LAT] 156 ms) to an extent that is comparable with LAP duration (F, G). Earliest activation of the left atrium in the septal region corresponds to -dV/dt max in lead V1 or V2 on surface electrocardiography (H). Reprinted with permission from Jadidi A, Müller-Edenborn B, Chen J, Keyl C, Weber R, Allgeier J, et al. The duration of the amplified sinus-P-wave identifies presence of left atrial low voltage substrate and predicts outcome after pulmonary vein isolation in patients with persistent atrial fibrillation. J Am Coll Cardiol EP 2018; 4: 531-543.

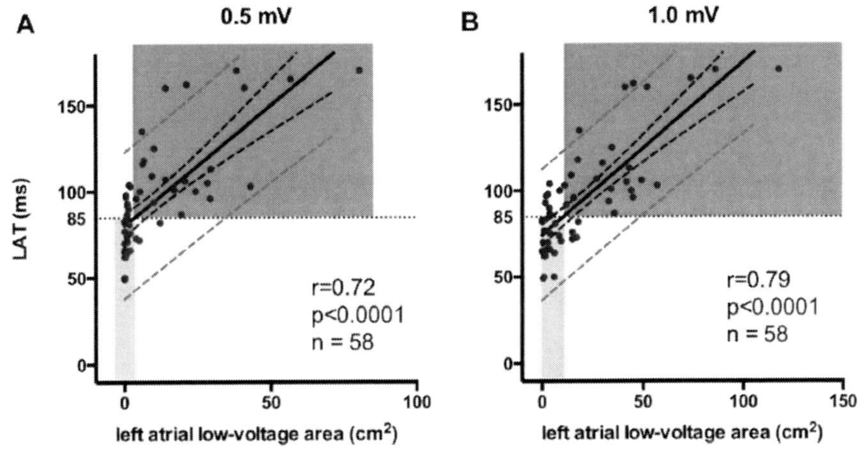

Figure 11. Correlation of Left Atrial Activation Time With Low Voltage Area. Seventy-two patients underwent left atrial (LA) mapping in sinus rhythm with a cutoff for low voltage of 0.5 mV (left) or 1.0 mV (right). LA activation time (LAT) was measured from the point of earliest activation in the left atrium (usually toward the anterior septum) to the point of latest activation in the region of the LA appendage. Linear regression analysis of LAT versus the different low-voltage cutoff values are shown. The best-fitting line of linear regression (black line), the 95% confidence bands (black dashed line), and the 95% prediction bands (gray dashed lines) are shown. Reprinted with permission from Jadidi A, Müller-Edenborn B, Chen J, Keyl C, Weber R, Allgeier J, et al. The duration of the amplified sinus-P-wave identifies presence of left atrial low voltage substrate and predicts outcome after pulmonary vein isolation in patients with persistent atrial fibrillation. J Am Coll Cardiol EP 2018; 4: 531-543.

Inter-atrial and intra-atrial conduction disturbances and other noninvasive index of atrial remodeling have been used in patients with paroxysmal and persistent atrial fibrillation [335-338]. Bayes de Luna A, et al. [335], in their electrocardiographic and vector-cardiographic study of interatrial conduction disturbances with left atrial retrograde activation, described an association of prolonged PWD with interatrial block and Bachmann bundle block with typical biphasic P-wave configuration in the inferior leads. Lin Y, et al. [338], observed in their study that the extent of left atrial low voltage substrate increases during the course of AF. They showed little to no left atrial low voltage substrate in early paroxysmal AF, and extensive atrial areas of low voltage substrate in long-standing or permanent AF. Platonov et al. [339] postulated that P-wave prolongation in AF may be due to conduction slowing and/or atrial enlargement. In this context, Jadidi AS, et al. demonstrated that regional left atrial low voltage

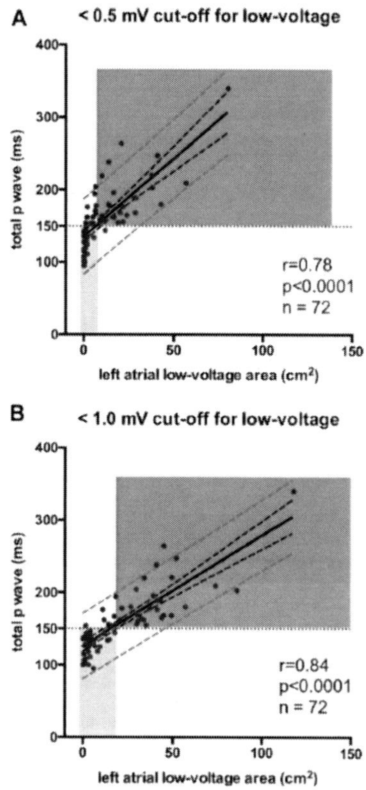

Figure 12. Correlation of Amplified P-Wave Duration on Surface 12-Lead-ECG to Extent of Left Atrial Low Voltage. Total P-wave duration was measured beginning at the earliest deflection from the baseline to the latest return to baseline in any lead of the 12-lead surface electrocardiogram. The extent of low voltage defined with cutoffs of < 0.5 mV (A) and < 1.0 mV (B) is shown with the best-fitting line of linear regression (black solid line), the 95% confidence bands (black dashed line), and the 95% prediction bands (gray dashed lines). ECG: electrocardiography. Reprinted with permission from Jadidi A, Müller-Edenborn B, Chen J, Keyl C, Weber R, Allgeier J, et al. The duration of the amplified sinus-P-wave identifies presence of left atrial low voltage substrate and predicts outcome after pulmonary vein isolation in patients with persistent atrial fibrillation. J Am Coll Cardiol EP 2018; 4: 531-543.

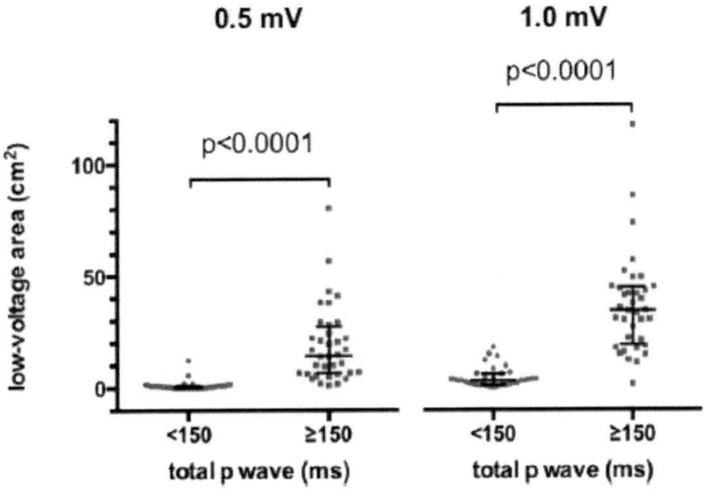

Figure 13. Extent of Left Atrial Low Voltage Stratified by P-Wave Duration. Extent of low-voltage substrate at 0.5 and 1.0 mV divided according to P-wave duration of < 150 or ≥ 150 ms. Whiskers depict mean ± SD. Reprinted with permission from Jadidi A, Müller-Edenborn B, Chen J, Keyl C, Weber R, Allgeier J, et al. The duration of the amplified sinus-P-wave identifies presence of left atrial low voltage substrate and predicts outcome after pulmonary vein isolation in patients with persistent atrial fibrillation. J Am Coll Cardiol EP 2018; 4: 531-543.

substrate as an electrophysiological correlate of local atrial fibrosis remodeling leads to conduction slowing, prolonged atrial activation time, and P-wave prolongation. Bayes de Luna A, et al. [335] suggested that fibrosis of the anteroseptal left atrial region accounts for the morphological changes of the P-wave, which is compatible with conduction slowing of the anterior interatrial connecting fibers (Bachmann's bundle). In line with those findings, conduction slowing as evidenced by increased PWD was later demonstrated to identify patients at risk for paroxysmal AF [340]. More recent studies have focused on the predictive value of the PWD in patients with AF for arrhythmia recurrences after PVI. These studies uniformly demonstrated that prolonged PWD was associated with a higher risk for arrhythmia recurrence in paroxysmal AF [341-345]. The reported cutoff values for PWD predicting AF recurrence post-pulmonary vein isolation, however, were highly variable and mostly arbitrarily chosen ranging from 120 to more than 165 ms [341-345]. A very recent meta-analysis of these studies concluded that a PWD greater than 149.5 ms in sinus rhythm was predictive for increased arrhythmia recurrences in patients with paroxysmal AF following pulmonary vein isolation [346]. Importantly, PWD was generally measured only after pulmonary vein isolation or cardioversion alone, as the respective studies focused on the potential left atrial reverse remodeling reflected by a decrease in PWD during the follow-up period [347, 348].

Recent studies revealed that arrhythmia freedom crucially depends on the presence or absence of left atrial structural abnormalities, as identified either by LGE-MRI [233, 248] or left atrial voltage mapping [284-287]. In the presence of significant left atrial low voltage substrate, pulmonary vein isolation plus additional ablation of target areas within the left atrial low voltage substrate was shown to improve arrhythmia freedom rates 1 year after the AF ablation procedure [284-287]. Quantification of LA fibrosis using delayed enhancement cardiac MRI was demonstrated to be feasible using specific MRI sequences. Although, LGE-MRI allows patient stratification prior to ablation, it is time-consuming, is expensive, requires intravenous injection of magnetic resonance contrast agents (gadolinium), and requires dedicated MRI sequence/fibrosis detection software that is likely unavailable at many hospitals. However, invasively measured left atrial activation time and P-wave duration on amplified and digitized 12-lead electrocardiography does not require extensive additional equipment and should be freely available to most cardiologists and electrophysiologists involved in the management of patients undergoing AF ablation. Patients with short duration of the P wave (< 150 ms) should be considered to have pulmonary vein–dependent persistent AF amenable to a PVI-only approach with high anticipated success rates using either radiofrequency or cryoballoon ablation. In contrast, patients with prolonged P wave duration of greater than 150 ms are likely to have persistent AF with additional, non–pulmonary vein–dependent foci, which likely requires more intensive atrial mapping and targeted ablation to achieve satisfying arrhythmia freedom rates. Future large-scale studies may answer if patients with prolonged PWD < 150 ms should receive oral anticoagulant therapy independent of AF history, to prevent cerebral and cardiac ischemic events.

Several studies performed in patients with persistent AF demonstrated higher arrhythmia freedom rates when pulmonary vein isolation plus additional ablation of left atrial low voltage substrate was performed [284-287]. Other studies involving simultaneous biatrial mapping of ongoing AF wavelets using basket catheters or body surface mapping using Cardio-Insight electrocardiographic imaging also reported higher arrhythmia freedom rates in patients with persistent AF compared with previous ablation or PVI-only strategies [349-353]. Large-scale prospective randomized multicenter studies like SOLVE-AF and DECAAF II investigating the best therapeutic approach in patients with persistent AF who have atrial low voltage substrate or delayed gadolinium enhancement are currently recruiting patients.

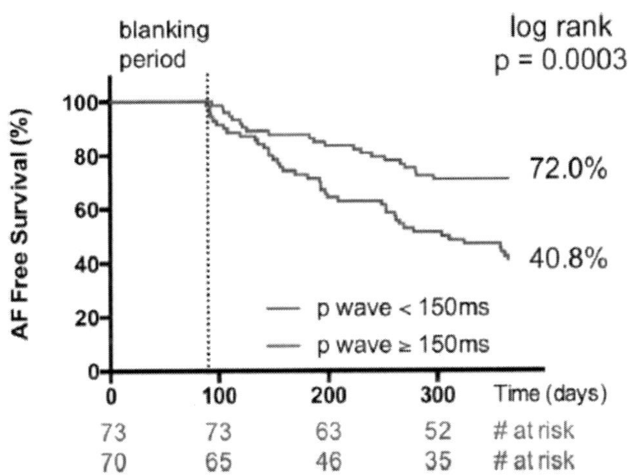

Figure 14. Arrhythmia Freedom Following Pulmonary Vein Isolation for Persistent Atrial Fibrillation Stratified According to P-Wave Duration. Kaplan-Meier curves are demonstrating the percentage of patients free from arrhythmia following pulmonary vein isolation for persistent atrial fibrillation at 1-year follow-up. The upper curve indicates patients with P-wave duration < 150 ms, and the lower curve demonstrates patients with P-wave duration ≥ 150 ms. Reprinted with permission from Jadidi A, Müller-Edenborn B, Chen J, Keyl C, Weber R, Allgeier J, et al. The duration of the amplified sinus-P-wave identifies presence of left atrial low voltage substrate and predicts outcome after pulmonary vein isolation in patients with persistent atrial fibrillation. J Am Coll Cardiol EP 2018; 4: 531-543.

Atrial fibrosis assessed noninvasively using late gadolinium-enhanced magnetic resonance imaging with current conventional techniques has pitfalls that should always be taken into account. Manual segmentation of the heart chambers and of the atrial scar tissue is time consuming and subject to inter-operator variability, particularly as image quality in AF is often poor. Therefore, the study of Yang G, et al. [280], is very interesting since it proposed a novel fully automatic pipeline to achieve accurate and objective segmentation of the heart from MRI Roadmap data, and of scar tissue within the heart from LGE-MRI data acquired in patients with AF. Their fully automatic pipeline uniquely combines: multi-atlas-based whole heart segmentation to determine the cardiac anatomy from an MRI Roadmap acquisition which is then mapped to LGE-MRI, and a super-pixel and supervised learning based approach to delineate the distribution and extent of atrial scarring in LGE-MRI. The authors compared the accuracy of the automatic analysis to manual ground truth segmentations in 37 patients with persistent long-standing AF. The authors found that both the multi-atlas whole heart segmentation and atrial scarring segmentations showed accurate delineations of cardiac anatomy (mean Dice = 89%) and atrial scarring (mean Dice = 79%), respectively, compared to the established ground truth from manual segmentation. In addition, compared to the ground truth, they obtained 88% segmentation accuracy, with 90% sensitivity and 79% specificity. The receiver operating characteristic analysis achieved an average area under the curve of 0.91. Therefore they concluded that compared with previously studied methods with manual interventions, the novel and innovative pipeline demonstrated comparable results, but was computed fully automatically. The proposed segmentation methods allow LGE-MRI to be used as an objective assessment tool for localization, visualization, and quantitation of atrial scarring and to guide ablation treatment [280].

Segmentation of the atrial scarring from LGE-MRI images is very challenging. The left atrium has a thin wall that measures only 2 mm. However, the difficulty is not only because the atrial scarring is difficult to distinguish in the thin LA wall but also because the image quality can be poor due to motion artifacts, noise contamination and contrast agent wash-out during the long acquisition. Moreover, the enhancement from the surrounding tissues and enhanced blood flow can result in increased false positives. In the study of Yang G, et al. [280] the fast and irregular heart rate in patients prior to ablation resulted in only 11 (65%) pre-ablation studies having good enough quality to be included in the study. Together with 26 (92%) post-ablation studies, the total number of datasets was limited to only 37 patients. The low number of pre-ablation studies included in their study is an indication of how difficult it is to scan patients in AF with LGE-MRI. However, developments in MRI acquisition strategies like beat-to-beat changes in inversion time and intelligent arrhythmia rejection schemes are likely to improve this difficulty. Nevertheless, their proposed pipeline has demonstrated an effective and efficient way to objectively segment and assess the atrial scarring. The authors have shown that both the multi-atlas-based whole heart segmentation and super-pixel classification-based atrial scarring segmentation have obtained satisfactory accuracy. Their study was performed using real clinical data. Hence, it may be useful to integrate their pipeline to clinical routines. The combination of patient-specific left atrial and pulmonary geometry model with an objective atrial scarring segmentation that can be rapidly obtained for individual AF patients without manual processing will certainly be beneficial.

The utilization of gadolinium has its side effects and has been challenged by recent reports. Gadolinium-based contrast agent is contraindicated in patients with severe renal impairment due to an increased risk of developing nephrogenic systemic fibrosis. In addition, there have been recent reports describing the retention of gadolinium in the body for up to several months after administration, even in patients with normal kidney function. This has led to the Federal Drugs Administration issuing a safety communication and while no direct association has been found between these deposits and adverse health effects in patients with normal kidney function, it has announced that a new class warning and safety measures will be required to appear in the labeling for gadolinium contrast agents used in MRI. Consideration should be given to the use of macrocyclic gadolinium agents, such as gadobutrol, rather than linear agents as they have reduced and shorter retention properties. The Federal Drugs Administration concludes that the benefit of all approved gadolinium contrast agents continues to outweigh potential risks and that healthcare professionals should not avoid or defer necessary examinations [354].

In the future, the combination of 3D EA voltage mapping and atrial substrate fibrosis ablation plus activation/phase mapping of rotors/re-entries might result in an additional increase in success rate. Almost nine years ago, LGE-MRI was introduced for detecting, quantifying, and localizing atrial fibrosis [271, 351]. In contrast to percutaneously invasive 3D EA voltage mapping, LGE-MRI looks attractive as a noninvasive, repeatable diagnostic tool. On the other hand, these cardiac MRI findings at this point in time require extensive MRI experience and the reproducibility is still under intensive investigation from other groups. The cardiac MRI quantification and localization of atrial fibrosis might also be used to guide individually tailored substrate elimination comparable to 3D EA voltage mapping guided substrate modification.

Conclusion

In conclusion, atrial fibrosis should be considered as a potential key factor in the mechanism of arrhythmia and in the management of AF. The development of atrial fibrosis is a multifactorial process resulting in complex neuro-humoral and cellular interactions. The consideration of atrial fibrosis for the therapeutic management of AF bears the potential to significantly improve AF understanding and clinical outcomes. LGE-MRI provides excellent advancement in the knowledge of the atrial substrate. It is a potent noninvasive diagnostic tool which allows for follow-up investigations without radiation exposure or risk from an invasive percutaneous procedure. Although, it is difficult to scan patients during AF with LGE-MRI, developments in MRI acquisition strategies like beat-to-beat changes in inversion time and intelligent arrhythmia rejection schemes are likely to improve this difficulty. Nevertheless, LGE-MRI techniques to assess LA fibrosis still require significant expertise; therefore, further technical improvements and more generalized imaging methods needs to be established.

There is a wide individual variation in the extent of left atrial fibrosis in patients with AF. Atrial fibrosis is the most important predictor of ablation failure beyond PV isolation. Voltage mapping as a tool for describing fibrotic changes is still under investigation. It is dependent on several biological and technological variables, and it still needs to be standardized. The atrial substrate fibrosis ablation is an effective rhythm control approach in AF patients despite durable PV isolation. The novel multi-atlas-based whole heart segmentation and super-pixel classification-based atrial scarring segmentation have obtained satisfactory accuracy. The combination of patient-specific left atrial and pulmonary geometry model with an objective manual processing atrial scarring segmentation will certainly be beneficial. All ablation strategies beyond PV isolation including fibrosis-guided ablation need to be confirmed and validated with respect to efficacy as well as safety in prospective multicenter randomized clinical studies. The SOLVE-AF and DECAAF II studies will probably help to improve the wide adoption of this important imaging tool.

REFERENCES

[1] Andrade, J; Khairy, P; Dobrev, D; Nattel, S. The clinical profile and pathophysiology of atrial fibrillation: relationships among clinical features, epidemiology, and mechanisms. *Circ Res*, 2014, 114, 1453-1468.

[2] Heijman, J; Algalarrondo, V; Voigt, N; et al. The value of basic research insights into atrial fibrillation mechanisms as a guide to therapeutic innovation: a critical analysis. *Cardiovasc Res*, 2016, 109, 467-479.

[3] Li, D; Fareh, S; Leung, TK; Nattel, S. Promotion of atrial fibrillation by heart failure in dogs: atrial remodeling of a different sort. *Circulation*, 1999, 100, 87-95.

[4] Zahid, S; Cochet, H; Boyle, PM; et al. Patient derived models link re-entrant driver localization in atrial fibrillation to fibrosis spatial pattern. *Cardiovasc Res*, 2016, 110, 443-454.

[5] Gal, P; Marrouche, NF. Magnetic resonance imaging of atrial fibrosis: redefining atrial fibrillation to a syndrome. *Eur Heart J*, 2017, 38, 14-19.

[6] Yue, L; Xie, J; Nattel, S. Molecular determinants of cardiac fibroblast electrical function and therapeutic implications for atrial fibrillation. *Cardiovasc Res*, 2011, 89, 744-753.

[7] Travers, JG; Kamal, FA; Robbins, J; Yutzey, KE; Blaxall, BC. Cardiac fibrosis: the fibroblast awakens. *Circ Res*, 2016, 118, 1021-1040.

[8] Burstein, B; Nattel, S. Atrial fibrosis: mechanisms and clinical relevance in atrial fibrillation. *J Am Coll Cardiol*, 2008, 51, 802-809.

[9] Weber, KT; Sun, Y; Bhattacharya, SK; Ahokas, RA; Gerling, IC. Myofibroblast-mediated mechanisms of pathological remodeling of the heart. *Nat Rev Cardiol*, 2013, 10, 15-26.

[10] Krul, SP; Berger, WR; Smit, NW; et al. Atrial fibrosis and conduction slowing in the left atrial appendage of patients undergoing thoracoscopic surgical pulmonary vein isolation for atrial fibrillation. *Circ Arrhythm Electrophysiol*, 2015, 8, 288-295.

[11] Hanna, N; Cardin, S; Leung, TK; Nattel, S. Differences in atrial versus ventricular remodeling in dogs with ventricular tachypacing-induced congestive heart failure. *Cardiovasc Res*, 2004, 63, 236-244.

[12] Burstein, B; Comtois, P; Michael, G; et al. Changes in connexin expression and the atrial fibrillation substrate in congestive heart failure. *Circ Res*, 2009, 105, 1213-1222.

[13] Nattel, S; Burstein, B; Dobrev, D. Atrial remodeling and atrial fibrillation: mechanisms and implications. *Circ Arrhythm Electrophysiol*, 2008, 1, 62-73.

[14] Lin, CS; Pan, CH. Regulatory mechanisms of atrial fibrotic remodeling in atrial fibrillation. *Cell Mol Life Sci*, 2008, 65, 1489-1508.

[15] Youn, JY; Zhang, J; Zhang, Y; et al. Oxidative stress in atrial fibrillation: an emerging role of NADPH oxidase. *J Mol Cell Cardiol*, 2013, 62, 72-79.

[16] Chen, Y; Surinkaew, S; Wu, CT; et al. JAK-STAT signaling and the atrial fibrillation-promoting fibrotic substrate: pathogenic role and possible therapeutic target. *Cardiovasc Res*, 2017, 113, 310-320.

[17] Carver, W; Goldsmith, EC. Regulation of tissue fibrosis by the biomechanical environment. *Biomed Res Int*, 2013, 2013, 101979.

[18] Shi, Y; Ducharme, A; Li, D; Gaspo, R; Nattel, S; Tardif, JC. Remodeling of atrial dimensions and emptying function in canine models of atrial fibrillation. *Cardiovasc Res*, 2001, 52, 217-225.

[19] Kawamura, M; Munetsugu, Y; Kawasaki, S; et al. Type III procollagen-N-peptide as a predictor of persistent atrial fibrillation recurrence after cardioversion. *Europace*, 2012, 14, 1719-1725.

[20] Rienks, M; Papageorgiou, AP; Frangogiannis, NG; Heymans, S. Myocardial extracellular matrix: an ever-changing and diverse entity. *Circ Res*, 2014, 114, 872-888.

[21] Halper, J; Kjaer, M. Basic components of connective tissues and extracellular matrix: elastin, fibrilin, fibulins, fibrinogen, fibronectin, laminin, tenascins and thrombospondins. *Adv Exp Med Biol*, 2014, 802, 31-47.

[22] Miragoli, M; Gaudesius, G; Rohr, S. Electrotonic modulation of cardiac impulse conduction by myofibroblasts. *Circ Res*, 2006, 98, 801-810.

[23] Zlochiver, S; Muñoz, V; Vikstrom, KL; Taffet, SM; Berenfeld, O; Jalife, J. Electrotonic myofibroblast-to-myocyte coupling increases propensity to reentrant arrhythmias in twodimensional cardiac monolayers. *Biophys J*, 2008, 95, 4469-4480.

[24] MacCannell, KA; Bazzazi, H; Chilton, L; Shibukawa, Y; Clark, RB; Giles, WR. A mathematical model of electrotonic interactions between ventricular myocytes and fibroblasts. *Biophys J*, 2007, 92, 4121-4132.

[25] Ashihara, T; Haraguchi, R; Nakazawa, K; et al. The role of fibroblasts in complex fractionated electrograms during persistent/permanent

atrial fibrillation: implications for electrogram-based catheter ablation. *Circ Res*, 2012, 110, 275-284.

[26] Aguilar, M; Qi, XY; Huang, H; Comtois, P; Nattel, S. Fibroblast electrical remodeling in heart failure and potential effects on atrial fibrillation. *Biophys J*, 2014, 107, 2444-2455.

[27] McDowell, KS; Vadakkumpadan, F; Blake, R; et al. Mechanistic inquiry into the role of tissue remodeling in fibrotic lesions in human atrial fibrillation. *Biophys J*, 2013, 104, 2764-2773.

[28] de Leeuw, N; Ruiter, DJ; Balk, AH. Histopathologic findings in explanted heart tissue from patients with end-stage idiopathic dilated cardiomyopathy. *Transpl Int*, 2001, 14, 299-306.

[29] Hughes, SE; McKenna, WJ. New insights into the pathology of inherited cardiomyopathy. *Heart*, 2005, 91, 257-264.

[30] O'Neill, JO; McCarthy, PM; Brunken, RC; et al. PET abnormalities in patients with nonischemic cardiomyopathy. *J Card Fail*, 2004, 10, 244-249.

[31] Knaapen, P; Boellaard, R; Gotte, MJ; et al. Perfusable tissue index as a potential marker of fibrosis in patients with idiopathic dilated cardiomyopathy. *J Nucl Med*, 2004, 45, 1299-1304.

[32] Ferrari, P; Bianchi, G. The genomics of cardiovascular disorders: therapeutic implications. *Drugs*, 2000, 59, 1025-1042.

[33] Ryoke, T; Gu, Y; Mao, L; et al. Progressive cardiac dysfunction and fibrosis in the cardiomyopathic hamster and effects of growth hormone and angiotensin-converting enzyme inhibition. *Circulation*, 1999, 100, 1734-1743.

[34] Heling, A; Zimmermann, R; Kostin, S; et al. Increased expression of cytoskeletal, linkage, and extracellular proteins in failing human myocardium. *Circ Res*, 2000, 86, 846-853.

[35] Izawa, H; Murohara, T; Nagata, K; et al. Mineralocorticoid receptor antagonism ameliorates left ventricular diastolic dysfunction and myocardial fibrosis in mildly symptomatic patients with idiopathic dilated cardiomyopathy: a pilot study. *Circulation*, 2005, 112, 2940-2945.

[36] Melenovsky, V; Hay, I; Fetics, BJ; et al. Functional impact of rate irregularity in patients with heart failure and atrial fibrillation receiving cardiac resynchronization therapy. *Eur Heart J*, 2005, 26, 705-711.

[37] MacKenna, DA; Omens, JH; MuCulloch, AD; Covell, JW. Contribution of collagen matrix to passive left ventricular mechanics in isolated rat hearts. *Am J Physiol*, 1994, 266, H1007-1018.

[38] Anderson, KR; Sutton, MG; Lie, JT. Histopathological types of cardiac fibrosis in myocardial disease. *J Pathol*, 1979, 128, 79-85.

[39] Schwarz, F; Mall, G; Zebe, H; et al. Quantitative morphologic findings of the myocardium in idiopathic dilated cardiomyopathy. *Am J Cardiol*, 1983, 51, 501-506.

[40] Unverferth, DV; Baker, PB; Swift, SE; et al. Extent of myocardial fibrosis and cellular hypertrophy in dilated cardiomyopathy. *Am J Cardiol*, 1986, 57, 816-820.

[41] Spach, MS; Miller, WT; Jr. Dolber, PC; et al. The functional role of structural complexities in the propagation of depolarization in the atrium of the dog: cardiac conduction disturbances due to discontinuities of effective axial resistivity. *Circ Res*, 1982, 50, 175-191.

[42] Spach, MS; Dolber, PC. Relating extracellular potentials and their derivatives to anisotropic propagation at a microscopic level in human cardiac muscle: evidence for electrical uncoupling of side-to-side fiber connections with increasing age. *Circ Res*, 1986, 58, 356-371.

[43] Fein, FS; Capasso, JM; Aronson, RS; et al. Combined renovascular hypertension and diabetes in rats: a new preparation of congestive cardiomyopathy. *Circulation*, 1984, 70, 318-330.

[44] Bakth, S; Arena, J; Lee, W; et al. Arrhythmia susceptibility and myocardial composition in diabetes: influence of physical conditioning. *J Clin Invest*, 1986, 77, 382-395.

[45] Anderson, KP; Walker, R; Urie, P; et al. Myocardial electrical propagation in patients with idiopathic dilated cardiomyopathy. *J Clin Invest*, 1993, 92, 122-140.

[46] de Bakker, JMT; van Capelle, FJL; Janse, MJ; et al. Fractionated electrograms in dilated cardiomyopathy: origin and relation to abnormal conduction. *J Am Coll Cardiol*, 1996, 27, 1071-1078.
[47] Lee, JJ; Kamjoo, K; Hough, D; et al. Reentrant wave fronts in Wiggers' stage II ventricular fibrillation: characteristics, and mechanisms of termination and spontaneous regeneration. *Circ Res*, 1996, 78, 660-675.
[48] Centurión, OA; Isomoto, S; Shimizu, A. Electrophysiological changes of the atrium in patients with lone paroxysmal atrial fibrillation. *J Atr Fibrillation*, 2010, 1(12), 656-662.
[49] Wu, TJ; Ong, JJ; Hwang, C; et al. Characteristics of wave fronts during ventricular fibrillation in human hearts with dilated cardiomyopathy: role of increased fibrosis in the generation of reentry. *J Am Coll Cardiol*, 1998, 32, 187-196.
[50] Centurión, OA. Atrial fibrillation in the Wolff-Parkinson-White syndrome. *J Atr Fibrillation*, 2011, 2, 899-915.
[51] Centurion, OA; Isomoto, S; Fukatani, M; Shimizu, A; Konoe, A; et al. Relationship between atrial conduction defects and fractionated atrial endocardial electrograms in patients with sick sinus syndrome. *Pace*, 1993, 16(10), 2022-2033.
[52] Centurion, OA; Shimizu, A; Isomoto, S; Konoe, A; Hirata, T; et al. Repetitive atrial firing and fragmented atrial activity elicited by extrastimuli in the sick sinus syndrome with and without abnormal atrial electrograms. *Am J Med Sci*, 1994, 307(4), 247-254.
[53] Centurion, OA; Fukatani, M; Konoe, A; Tanigawa, M; Shimizu, A; et al. Different distribution of abnormal endocardial electrograms within the right atrium in patients with sick sinus syndrome. *Br Heart J*, 1992, 68(6), 596-600.
[54] Centurión, OA; Isomoto, S; Shimizu, A; et al. The effects of aging on atrial endocardial electrograms in patients with paroxysmal atrial fibrillation. *Clin Cardiol*, 2003, 26, 435-438.
[55] Centurión, OA; Shimizu, A; Isomoto, S; et al. Influence of advancing age on fractionated right atrial endocardial electrograms. *Am J Cardiol*, 2005, 96, 239-242.

[56] Centurión, OA; Shimizu, A; Isomoto, S; Konoe, A. Mechanisms for the genesis of paroxysmal atrial fibrillation in the Wolf-Parkinson-White syndrome: Intrinsic atrial muscle vulnerability vs. electrophysiological properties of the accessory pathway. *Europace*, 2008, 10, 294-302.

[57] Shimizu, A; Centurión, OA. Electrophysiological properties of the human atrial fibrillation. *Cardiovasc Res*, 2002, 54(2), 302-314.

[58] Centurión, OA; et al. Electrophysiological changes of the atrium in patients with lone paroxysmal atrial fibrillation. *J Atr Fibrillation*, 2010, 3(1), 232.

[59] Centurión, OA. Age-related electrophysiological changes of the atrial myocardium in patients with paroxysmal atrial fibrillation. *J Cardiol Curr Res*, 2015, 3(6), 00121.

[60] Centurión, OA; et al. Electrophysiological Abnormalities of the Atrial Myocardium and the Rubenstein Clinical Classification of Patients with Sinus Node Dysfunction. *EC Cardiology*, 2018, 5(11), 846-857.

[61] Dillon, SM; Allessie, MA; Ursell, PC; Wit, AL. Influences of anisotropic tissue structure on reentrant circuits in the epicardial border zone of subacute canine infarcts. *Circ Res*, 1988, 63, 182-206.

[62] Ursell, PC; Gardner, PI; Albala, A; Fenoglio, JJ; Wit, AL. Structural and electrophysiological changes in the epicardial border zone and canine myocardial infarcts during infarct healing. *Circ Res*, 1985, 56, 436-451.

[63] Pogwizd, SM; Hoyt, RH; Saffitz, JE; et al. Reentrant and focal mechanisms underlying ventricular tachycardia in the human heart. *Circulation*, 1992, 86, 1872-1887.

[64] Delgado, C; Steinhaus, B; Delmar, M; Chialvo, DR; Jalife, J. Directional differences in excitability and margin of safety for propagation in sheep ventricular epicardial muscle. *Circ Res*, 1990, 67, 97-110.

[65] Nazer, B; Gerstenfeld, E. Catheter ablation of ventricular tachycardia in patients with post-infarction cardiomyopathy. *Korean Circ J*, 2014, 44(4), 210-217.

[66] Tung, R; Boyle, NG; Shivkumar, K. Catheter ablation of ventricular tachycardia. *Circulation.*, 2011, 123(20), 2284-2288.

[67] Arbustini, E; Narula, N; Dec, GW; et al. The MOGE(S) classification for a phenotype-genotype nomenclature of cardiomyopathy: endorsed by the World Heart Federation. *J Am Coll Cardiol*, 2013, 62, 2046-72.

[68] Goldberger, JJ; Cain, ME; Hohnloser, SH; et al. American Heart Association/American College of Cardiology Foundation/Heart Rhythm Society scientific statement on noninvasive risk stratification techniques for identifying patients at risk for sudden cardiac death. *Circulation*, 2008, 118, 1497-518.

[69] Bardy, GH; Lee, KL; Mark, DB; et al. Amiodarone or an implantable cardioverter-defibrillator for congestive heart failure. *N Engl J Med*, 2005, 352, 225-237.

[70] Kadish, A; Dyer, A; Daubert, JP; et al. Prophylactic defibrillator implantation in patients with nonischemic dilated cardiomyopathy. *N Engl J Med*, 2004, 350, 2151-2158.

[71] Epstein, AE; DiMarco, JP; Ellenbogen, KA; et al. 2012 ACCF/AHA/HRS focused update incorporated into the ACCF/ AHA/HRS 2008 guidelines for device-based therapy of cardiac rhythm abnormalities: a report of the American College of Cardiology Foundation/American Heart Association Task Force on Practice Guidelines and the Heart Rhythm Society. *J Am Coll Cardiol*, 2013, 61, e6-e75.

[72] Hartikainen, JE; Malik, M; Staunton, A; Poloniecki, J; Camm, AJ. Distinction between arrhythmic and nonarrhythmic death after acute myocardial infarction based on heart rate variability, signal-averaged electrocardiogram, ventricular arrhythmias and left ventricular ejection fraction. *J Am Coll Cardiol*, 1996, 28, 296-304.

[73] Buxton, AE; Lee, KL; Hafley, GE; et al. Limitations of ejection fraction for prediction of sudden risk death in patients with coronary artery disease: lessons from the MUSTT study. *J Am Coll Cardiol*, 2007, 50, 1150-1157.

[74] Ezekowitz, JA; Rowe, BH; Dryden, DM; et al. Systematic review: implantable cardioverter defibrillators for adults with left ventricular systolic dysfunction. *Ann Intern Med*, 2007, 147, 251-262.

[75] Bello, D; Fieno, DS; Kim, RJ; et al. Infarct morphology identifies patients with substrate for sustained ventricular tachycardia. *J Am Coll Cardiol*, 2005, 45, 1104-1108.

[76] Bogun, FM; Desjardins, B; Good, E; et al. Delayed enhanced magnetic resonance imaging in nonischemic cardiomyopathy: utility for identifying the ventricular arrhythmia substrate. *J Am Coll Cardiol*, 2009, 53, 1138-1145.

[77] Roes, SD; Borleffs, CJ; van der Geest, RJ; et al. Infarct tissue heterogeneity assessed with contrast enhanced MRI predicts spontaneous ventricular arrhythmias in patients with ischemic cardiomyopathy and implantable cardioverter-defibrillator. *Circ Cardiovasc Imaging*, 2009, 2, 183-190.

[78] Gao, P; Yee, R; Gula, L; et al. Prediction of arrhythmic events in ischemic and dilated cardiomyopathy patients referred for implantable cardiac defibrillator: evaluation of multiple scar quantification measures for late gadolinium enhancement magnetic resonance imaging. *Circ Cardiovasc Imaging*, 2012, 5, 448-456.

[79] Klem, I; Weinsaft, JW; Bahnson, TD; et al. Assessment of myocardial scarring improves risk stratification in patients evaluated for cardiac defibrillator implantation. *J Am Coll Cardiol*, 2012, 60, 408-420.

[80] Gulati, A; Jabbour, A; Ismail, TF; et al. Association of fibrosis with mortality and sudden cardiac death in patients with nonischemic dilated cardiomyopathy. *JAMA*, 2013, 309, 896-908.

[81] Neilan, TG; Coelho-Filho, OR; Danik, SB; et al. CMR quantification of myocardial scar provides additive prognostic information in nonischemic cardiomyopathy. *J Am Coll Cardiol Img*, 2013, 6(9), 944-954.

[82] Machii, M; Satoh, H; Shiraki, K; et al. Distribution of late gadolinium enhancement in end-stage hypertrophic cardiomyopathy and dilated cardiomyopathy: differential diagnosis and prediction of cardiac outcome. *Magn Reson Imaging*, 2014, 32, 118-124.

[83] Masci, PG; Doulaptsis, C; Bertella, E; et al. Incremental prognostic value of myocardial fibrosis in patients with non-ischemic cardiomyopathy without congestive heart failure. *Circ Heart Fail*, 2014, 7, 448-456.

[84] Nabeta, T; Inomata, T; Iida, Y; et al. Baseline cardiac magnetic resonance imaging versus baseline endomyocardial biopsy for the prediction of left ventricular reverse remodeling and prognosis in response to therapy in patients with idiopathic dilated cardiomyopathy. *Heart Vessels*, 2014, 29, 784-792.

[85] Poyhonen, P; Kivisto, S; Holmstrom, M; Hanninen, H. Quantifying late gadolinium enhancement on CMR provides additional prognostic information in early risk-stratification of nonischemic cardio-myopathy: a cohort study. *BMC Cardiovasc Disord*, 2014, 14, 110.

[86] Rodriguez-Capitan, J; Garcia-Pinilla, JM; Ruiz-Zamora, I; et al. Long-term prognostic value of late gadolinium enhancement in a cohort of patients with nonischemic dilated cardiomyopathy. *Int J Cardiol*, 2014, 177, 17-19.

[87] Halliday, BP; Gulati, A; Ali, A; et al. Association between midwall late gadolinium enhancement and sudden cardiac death in patients with dilated cardiomyopathy and mild and moderate left ventricular systolic dysfunction. *Circulation*, 2017, 135, 2106-2115.

[88] Yamada, T; Hirashiki, A; Okumura, T; et al. Prognostic impact of combined late gadolinium enhancement on cardiovascular magnetic resonance and peak oxygen consumption in ambulatory patients with nonischemic dilated cardiomyopathy. *J Card Fail*, 2014, 20, 825-832.

[89] Chimura, M; Kiuchi, K; Okajima, K; et al. Distribution of ventricular fibrosis associated with life threatening ventricular tachyarrhythmias in patients with nonischemic dilated cardiomyopathy. *J Cardiovasc Electrophysiol*, 2015, 26, 1239-1246.

[90] Piers, SR; Everaerts, K; van der Geest, RJ; et al. Myocardial scar predicts monomorphic ventricular tachycardia but not polymorphic ventricular tachycardia or ventricular fibrillation in nonischemic dilated cardiomyopathy. *Heart Rhythm*, 2015, 12, 2106-2114.

[91] Tateishi, E; Noguchi, T; Goto, Y; et al. Prognostic impact of blood pressure response plus gadolinium enhancement in dilated cardiomyopathy. *Heart*, 2015, 101, 774-780.

[92] Park, S; Choi, BW; Rim, SJ; et al. Delayed hyperenhancement magnetic resonance imaging is useful in predicting functional recovery of nonischemic left ventricular systolic dysfunction. *J Card Fail*, 2006, 12, 93-99.

[93] Gaztanaga, J; Paruchuri, V; Elias, E; et al. Prognostic value of late gadolinium enhancement in nonischemic cardiomyopathy. *Am J Cardiol*, 2016, 118, 1063-1068.

[94] Hu, DJ; Xu, J; Du, W; Zhang, JX; Zhong, M; Zhou, YN. Cardiac magnetic resonance and galectin-3 level as predictors of prognostic outcomes for non-ischemic cardiomyopathy patients. *Int J Cardiovasc Imaging*, 2016, 32, 1725-1733.

[95] Mikami, Y; Cornhill, A; Heydari, B; et al. Objective criteria for septal fibrosis in non-ischemic dilated cardiomyopathy: validation for the prediction of future cardiovascular events. *J Cardiovasc Magn Reson*, 2016, 18, 82.

[96] Puntmann, VO; Carr-White, G; Jabbour, A; et al. T1-mapping and outcome in nonischemic cardiomyopathy: all-cause mortality and heart failure. *J Am Coll Cardiol Img*, 2016, 9, 40-50.

[97] Shin, DG; Lee, HJ; Park, J; et al. Pattern of late gadolinium enhancement predicts arrhythmic events in patients with non-ischemic cardiomyopathy. *Int J Cardiol*, 2016, 222, 9–15.

[98] Tachi, M; Amano, Y; Inui, K; et al. Relationship of postcontrast myocardial T1 value and delayed enhancement to reduced cardiac function and serious arrhythmia in dilated cardiomyopathy with left ventricular ejection fraction less than 35%. *Acta Radiol*, 2016, 57, 430-436.

[99] Marume, K; Noguchi, T; Tateishi, E; Morita, Y; Kamakura, T; Ishibashi, K; et al. Mortality and sudden cardiac death risk stratification using the noninvasive combination of wide QRS duaration and late gadolinium enhancement in idiopathic dilated

cardiomyopathy. *Circ Arrhythm Electrophysiol*, 2018, 11, e006233. doi: 10.1161/CIRCEP.117.006233.

[100] Mann, DL; Bristow, MR. Mechanisms and models in heart failure: the biomechanical model and beyond. *Circulation*, 2005, 111, 2837-2849.

[101] Iles, LM; Ellims, AH; Llewellyn, H; et al. Histological validation of cardiac magnetic resonance analysis of regional and diffuse interstitial myocardial fibrosis. *Eur Heart J Cardiovasc Imaging*, 2015, 16, 14-22.

[102] Schmidt, A; Azevedo, CF; Cheng, A; et al. Infarct tissue heterogeneity by magnetic resonance imaging identifies enhanced cardiac arrhythmias susceptibility in patients with left ventricular dysfunction. *Circulation*, 2007, 115, 2006-2014.

[103] Perez-David, E; Arenal, A; Rubio-Guivernau, JL; et al. Noninvasive identification of ventricular tachycardia-related conduction channel using contrast-enhanced magnetic resonance imaging in patients with chronic myocardial infarction: comparison of signal intensity scar mapping and endocardial voltage mapping. *J Am Coll Cardiol*, 2011, 57, 184-194.

[104] Kwong, RY; Farzaneh-Far, A. Measuring myocardial scar by CMR. *J Am Coll Cardiol Img*, 2011, 4, 157-160.

[105] Disertori, M; Quintarelli, S; Mazzola, S; Favalli, V; Narula, N; Arbustini, E. The need to modify patient selection to improve the benefits of implantable cardioverter-defibrillator for primary prevention of sudden death in non-ischaemic dilated cardiomyopathy. *Europace*, 2013, 15, 1693-1701.

[106] Assomull, RG; Prasad, SK; Lyne, J; et al. Cardiovascular magnetic resonance, fibrosis, and prognosis in dilated cardiomyopathy. *J Am Coll Cardiol*, 2006, 48, 1977-1985.

[107] Wu, KC; Weiss, RG; Thiemann, DR; et al. Late gadolinium enhancement by cardiovascular magnetic resonance heralds an adverse prognosis in nonischemic cardiomyopathy. *J Am Coll Cardiol*, 2008, 51, 2414-2421.

[108] Hsia, H; Marchlinski, F. Characterization of the electroanatomic substrate for monomorphic ventricular tachycardia in patients with nonischemic cardiomyopathy. *Pacing Clin Electrophysiol*, 2002, 25, 1114-1127.

[109] Wu, TJ; Ong, JJC; Hwang, C; et al. Characteristics of wave fronts during ventricular fibrillation in human hearts with dilated cardiomyopathy: role of increased fibrosis in the generation of reentry. *J Am Coll Cardiol*, 1998, 32, 187-196.

[110] Nazarian, S; Bluemke, DA; Lardo, AC; et al. Magnetic resonance assessment of the substrate for inducible ventricular tachycardia in nonischemic cardiomyopathy. *Circulation*, 2005, 112, 2821-2825.

[111] Moon, JCC; Reed, E; Sheppard, MN; et al. The histologic basis of late gadolinium enhancement cardiovascular magnetic resonance in hypertrophic cardiomyopathy. *J Am Coll Cardiol*, 2004, 43, 2260-2264.

[112] McCrohon, JA; Moon, JC; Prasad, SK; et al. Differentiation of heart failure related to dilated cardiomyopathy and coronary artery disease using gadolinium-enhanced cardiovascular magnetic resonance. *Circulation*, 2003, 108, 54-59.

[113] Taylor, AJ; Al-Saadi, N; Abdel-Aty, H; Schulz-Menger, J; Messroghli, DR; Friedrich, MG. Detection of acutely impaired microvascular reperfusion after infarct angioplasty with magnetic resonance imaging. *Circulation*, 2004, 109, 2080-2085.

[114] Wijffels, MC; Kirchhof, CJ; Dorland, R; Allessie, MA. Atrial fibrillation begets atrial fibrillation. A study in awake chronically instrumented goats. *Circulation*, 1995, 92, 1954-1968.

[115] Ausma, J; Wijffels, M; Thone, F; Wouters, L; Allessie, M; Borgers, M. Structural changes of atrial myocardium due to sustained atrial fibrillation in the goat. *Circulation*, 1997, 96, 3157-3163.

[116] Burstein, B; Qi, XY; Yeh, YH; Calderone, A; Nattel, S. Atrial cardiomyocyte tachycardia alters cardiac fibroblast function: a novel consideration in atrial remodeling. *Cardiovasc Res*, 2007, 76, 442-452.

[117] Li, D; Fareh, S; Leung, TK; Nattel, S. Promotion of atrial fibrillation by heart failure in dogs: atrial remodeling of a different sort. *Circulation*, 1999, 100, 87-95.

[118] Tilz, RR; Rillig, A; Thum, AM; et al. Catheter ablation of long-standing persistent atrial fibrillation: 5-year outcomes of the Hamburg Sequential Ablation Strategy. *J Am Coll Cardiol*, 2012, 60, 1921-1929.

[119] Kirchhof, P; Benussi, S; Kotecha, D; et al. 2016 ESC guidelines for the management of atrial fibrillation developed in collaboration with EACTS. *Eur Heart J*, 2016, 37, 2893-2962.

[120] Goette, A; Kalman, JM; Aguinaga, L; et al. EHRA/ HRS/ APHRS/SOLAECE expert consensus on atrial cardiomyopathies: definition, characterization, and clinical implication. *Heart Rhythm*, 2017, 14, e3–40.

[121] Cochet, H; Mouries, A; Nivet, H; et al. Age, atrial fibrillation, and structural heart disease are the main determinants of left atrial fibrosis detected by delayed-enhanced magnetic resonance imaging in a general cardiology population. *J Cardiovasc Electrophysiol*, 2015, 26, 484-492.

[122] Mahnkopf, C; Badger, TJ; Burgon, NS; et al. Evaluation of the left atrial substrate in patients with lone atrial fibrillation using delayed enhanced MRI: implications for disease progression and response to catheter ablation. *Heart Rhythm*, 2010, 7, 1475-1481.

[123] Kuppahally, SS; Akoum, N; Badger, TJ; et al. Echocardiographic left atrial reverse remodeling after catheter ablation of atrial fibrillation is predicted by preablation delayed enhancement of left atrium by magnetic resonance imaging. *Am Heart J*, 2010, 160, 877-884.

[124] Moe, CK. On the multiple wavelet hypothesis of atrial fibrillation. *Arch Int Pharmacodyn Ther*, 1962, 140, 183-188.

[125] Moe, GK; Abildskov, IA. Atrial fibrillation as a self sustaining arrhythmia independent of focal discharge. *Am Heart J*, 1959, 58, 59-70.

[126] Moe, CK; Rheinboldt, WC. Abildskov IA. A computer model of atrial fibrillation. *Am Heart J*, 1964, 67, 200-220.

[127] Wijffels, MC; Kirchhof, CJ; Dorland, R; Allessie, MA. Atrial fibrillation begets atrial fibrillation. A study in awake chronically instrumented goats. *Circulation.*, 1995, 92, 1954-1968.

[128] Allessie, MA; Konings, K; Kirchhof, CJ; Wijffels, M. Electrophysiologic mechanisms of perpetuation of atrial fibrillation. *Am J Cardiol.*, 1996, 77, 10A-23A.

[129] Allessie, MA; Kirchhof, CJ; Konings, KT. Unraveling the electrical mysteries of atrial fibrillation. *Eur Heart J.*, 1996, 17 Suppl C, 2-9.

[130] Li, D; Fareh, S; Leung, TK; Nattel, S. Promotion of atrial fibrillation by heart failure in dogs: atrial remodeling of a different sort. *Circulation*, 1999, 100, 87–95.

[131] Mary-Rabine, L; Albert, A; Pham, TD; et al. The relationship of human atrial cellular electrophysiology to clinical function and ultrastructure. *Circ Res.*, 1983, 52, 188–199.

[132] Elvan, A; Huang, X; Pressler, M; et al. Radiofrequency catheter ablation of the atria eliminates pacing induced sustained atrial fibrillation and reduces connexion 43 in dogs. *Circulation.*, 1997, 96, 1675–1685.

[133] van der Velden, HMW; van Kempen, MJA; Wijffels, MCEF; et al. Altered pattern of connexin40 distribution in persistent atrial fibrillation in the goat. *J Cardiovasc Electrophysiol.*, 1998, 9, 596–607.

[134] Verheule, S; Sato, T; Everett, T; et al. Increased vulnerability to atrial fibrillation in transgenic mice with selective atrial fibrosis caused by overexpression of TGF-beta1. *Circ Res*, 2004, 94, 1458–65.

[135] Xiao, HD; Fuchs, S; Campbell, DJ; et al. Mice with cardiac-restricted angiotensin-converting enzyme (ACE) have atrial enlargement, cardiac arrhythmia, and sudden death. *Am J Pathol*, 2004, 165, 1019 –32.

[136] Lin, CS; Lai, LP; Lin, JL; et al. Increased expression of extracellular matrix proteins in rapid atrial pacing-induced atrial fibrillation. *HeartRhythm*, 2007, 4, 938–49.

[137] Calkins, H; Kuck, KH; Cappato, R; et al. 2012 HRS/EHRA/ECAS expert consensus statement on catheter and surgical ablation of atrial fibrillation: recommendations for patient selection, procedural

techniques, patient management and follow-up, definitions, endpoints, and research trial design: a report of the Heart Rhythm Society (HRS) Task Force on Catheter and Surgical Ablation of Atrial Fibrillation. *Heart Rhythm*, 2012, 9, 632-696.e21.

[138] Marrouche, NF; Wilber, D; Hindricks, G; et al. Association of atrial tissue fibrosis identified by delayed enhancement MRI and atrial fibrillation catheter ablation: the DECAAF study. *JAMA*, 2014, 311, 498-506.

[139] Han, FT; Akoum, N; Marrouche, N. Value of magnetic resonance imaging in guiding atrial fibrillation management. *Can J Cardiol*, 2013, 29, 1194-1202.

[140] Akoum, N; Daccarett, M; McGann, C; et al. Atrial fibrosis helps select the appropriate patient and strategy in catheter ablation of atrial fibrillation: a DE-MRI guided approach. *J Cardiovasc Electrophysiol*, 2011, 22, 16-22.

[141] Akoum, N; Wilber, D; Hindricks, G; et al. MRI assessment of ablation-induced scarring in atrial fibrillation: analysis from the DECAAF study. *J Cardiovasc Electrophysiol*, 2015, 26, 473-480.

[142] Elliott, AD; Mahajan, R; Pathak, RK; Lau, DH; Sanders, P. Exercise training and atrial fibrillation: further evidence for the importance of lifestyle change. *Circulation*, 2016, 133, 457-459.

[143] Pathak, RK; Middeldorp, ME; Lau, DH; et al. Aggressive risk factor reduction study for atrial fibrillation and implications for the outcome of ablation: the ARREST-AF cohort study. *J Am Coll Cardiol*, 2014, 64, 2222-2231.

[144] Pedersen, OD; Bagger, H; Kober, L; Torp-Pedersen, C. Trandolapril reduces the incidence of atrial fibrillation after acute myocardial infarction in patients with left ventricular dysfunction. *Circulation*, 1999, 100, 376-380.

[145] Li, D; Shinagawa, K; Pang, L; et al. Effects of angiotensin-converting enzyme inhibition on the development of the atrial fibrillation substrate in dogs with ventricular tachypacing-induced congestive heart failure. *Circulation*, 2001, 104, 2608-2614.

[146] Daccarett, M; Badger, TJ; Akoum, N; et al. Association of left atrial fibrosis detected by delayed-enhancement magnetic resonance imaging and the risk of stroke in patients with atrial fibrillation. *J Am Coll Cardiol*, 2011, 57, 831-838.

[147] Lip, GY; Nieuwlaat, R; Pisters, R; Lane, DA; Crijns, HJ. Refining clinical risk stratification for predicting stroke and thromboembolism in atrial fibrillation using a novel risk factor-based approach: the Euro Heart Survey on Atrial Fibrillation. *Chest*, 2010, 137, 263-272.

[148] Lane, DA; Lip, GY. Use of the CHA(2)DS(2)-VASc and HAS-BLED scores to aid decision making for thromboprophylaxis in nonvalvular atrial fibrillation. *Circulation*, 2012, 126, 860-865.

[149] Healey, JS; Connolly, SJ; Gold, MR; et al. Subclinical atrial fibrillation and the risk of stroke. *N Engl J Med*, 2012, 366, 120-129.

[150] Disertori, M; Quintarelli, S; Grasso, M; et al. Autosomal recessive atrial dilated cardiomyopathy with standstill evolution associated with mutation of Natriuretic Peptide Precursor A. *Circ Cardiovasc Genet*, 2013, 6, 27-36.

[151] Spronk, HM; De Jong, AM; Verheule, S; et al. Hypercoagulability causes atrial fibrosis and promotes atrial fibrillation. *Eur Heart J*, 2017, 38, 38-50.

[152] Erdogan, O. Risk assessment and therapy decision in patients at low risk for stroke: CHA2DS2-VASc vs. CHADS2? *Eur Heart J*, 2013, 34, 168-169.

[153] Mackenzie, J. Diseases of the Heart. 3rd edition. London, UK: Oxford Medical Publications, 1914.

[154] Anter, E; Jessup, M; Callans, DJ. Atrial fibrillation and heart failure: treatment considerations for a dual epidemic. *Circulation*, 2009, 119, 2516-2525.

[155] Kotecha, D; Piccini, JP. Atrial fibrillation in heart failure: what should we do? *Eur Heart J*, 2015, 36, 3250-3257.

[156] Stewart, S; Hart, CL; Hole, DJ; McMurray, JJ. A population-based study of the long-term risks associated with atrial fibrillation: 20-year follow-up of the Renfrew/Paisley study. *Am J Med*, 2002, 113, 359-364.

[157] Maisel, WH; Stevenson, LW. Atrial fibrillation in heart failure: epidemiology, pathophysiology, and rationale for therapy. *Am J Cardiol*, 2003, 91, 2D-8D.

[158] Ehrlich, JR; Nattel, S; Hohnloser, SH. Atrial fibrillation and congestive heart failure: specific considerations at the intersection of two common and important cardiac disease sets. *J Cardiovasc Electrophysiol*, 2002, 13, 399-405.

[159] Nattel, S; Burstein, B; Dobrev, D. Atrial remodeling and atrial fibrillation: mechanisms and implications. *Circ Arrhythm Electrophysiol*, 2008, 1, 62-73.

[160] Wijesurendra, RS; Liu, A; Eichhorn, C; et al. Lone atrial fibrillation is associated with impaired left ventricular energetics that persists despite successful catheter ablation. *Circulation*, 2016, 134, 1068-1081.

[161] Wakili, R; Voigt, N; Kaab, S; Dobrev, D; Nattel, S. Recent advances in the molecular pathophysiology of atrial fibrillation. *J Clin Invest*, 2011, 121, 2955-2968.

[162] Akkaya, M; Higuchi, K; Koopmann, M; et al. Higher degree of left atrial structural remodeling in patients with atrial fibrillation and left ventricular systolic dysfunction. *J Cardiovasc Electrophysiol*, 2013, 24, 485-491.

[163] Machino-Ohtsuka, T; Seo, Y; Ishizu, T; et al. Significant improvement of left atrial and left atrial appendage function after catheter ablation for persistent atrial fibrillation. *Circ J*, 2013, 77, 1695-1704.

[164] Gelsomino, S; Luca, F; Rao, CM; et al. Improvement of left atrial function and left atrial reverse remodeling after surgical treatment of atrial fibrillation. *Ann Cardiothorac Surg*, 2014, 3, 70-74.

[165] Gal, P; Pacchia, C; Morris, A; et al. Ablation scar recovery is significantly stronger in atrial fibrillation free patients (abstr P258). Poster Session: "Best Abstracts". *Europace*, 2015, 17 Suppl 3, iii20-29.

[166] Badger, TJ; Daccarett, M; Akoum, NW; et al. Evaluation of left atrial lesions after initial and repeat atrial fibrillation ablation: lessons

learned from delayed-enhancement MRI in repeat ablation procedures. *Circ Arrhythm Electrophysiol*, 2010, 3, 249-259.

[167] Kottkamp, H. Human atrial fibrillation substrate: towards a specific fibrotic atrial cardiomyopathy. *Eur Heart J*, 2013, 34, 2731-2738.

[168] Callans, DJ; Ren, JF; Michele, J; Marchlinski, FE; Dillon, SM. Electroanatomic left ventricular mapping in the porcine model of healed anterior myocardial infarction. Correlation with intra-cardiac echocardiography and pathological analysis. *Circulation*, 1999, 100, 1744-1750.

[169] Jadidi, AS; Cochet, H; Shah, AJ; et al. Inverse relationship between fractionated electrograms and atrial fibrosis in persistent atrial fibrillation combined magnetic resonance imaging and high density mapping. *J Am Coll Cardiol*, 2013, 62, 802-812.

[170] Kirubakaran, S; Chowdhury, RA; Hall, MC; Patel, PM; Garratt, CJ; Peters, NS. Fractionation of electrograms is caused by colocalized conduction block and connexin disorganization in the absence of fibrosis as AF becomes persistent in the goat model. *Heart Rhythm*, 2015, 12, 397-408.

[171] Harrison, JL; Jensen, HK; Peel, SA; et al. Cardiac magnetic resonance and electroanatomical mapping of acute and chronic atrial ablation injury: a histological validation study. *Eur Heart J*, 2014, 35, 1486-1495.

[172] Malcolme-Lawes, LC; Juli, C; Karim, R; et al. Automated analysis of atrial late gadolinium enhancement imaging that correlates with endocardial voltage and clinical outcomes: a 2-center study. *Heart Rhythm*, 2013, 10, 1184-1191.

[173] Jais, P; Shah, DC; Haissaguerre, M; et al. Mapping and ablation of left atrial flutters. *Circulation*, 2000, 101, 2928-2934.

[174] Watanabe, Y; Nakano, Y; Hidaka, T; et al. Mechanical and substrate abnormalities of the left atrium assessed by 3-dimensional speckle tracking echocardiography and electroanatomic mapping system in patients with paroxysmal atrial fibrillation. *Heart Rhythm*, 2015, 12, 490-497.

[175] Tanaka, K; Zlochiver, S; Vikstrom, KL; Yamazaki, M; et al. Spatial distribution of fibrosis governs fibrillation wave dynamics in the posterior left atrium during heart failure. *Circ Res.*, 2007, 101, 839-847.

[176] Haissaguerre, M; Jais, P; Shah, DC; Gencel, L; et al. Right and left atrial radiofrequency catheter therapy of paroxysmal atrial fibrillation. *J Cardiovasc Electrophysiol.*, 1996, 7, 1132-1144.

[177] Jais, P; Shah, DC; Takahashi, A; Hocini, M; et al. Long-term follow-up after right atrial radiofrequency catheter treatment of paroxysmal atrial fibrillation. *Pacing Clin Electrophysiol.*, 1998, 21, 2533-2538.

[178] Natale, A; Leonelli, F; Beheiry, S; Newby, K; et al. Catheter ablation approach on the right side only for paroxysmal atrial fibrillation therapy: long-term results. *Pacing Clin Electrophysiol.*, 2000, 23, 224-233.

[179] Jais, P; Shah, DC; Haissaguerre, M; Takahashi, A; et al. Efficacy and safety of septal and left-atrial linear ablation for atrial fibrillation. *Am J Cardiol.*, 1999, 84, 139R-146R.

[180] Haissaguerre, M; Jais, P; Shah, DC; Takahashi, A; et al. Spontaneous initiation of atrial fibrillation by ectopic beats originating in the pulmonary veins. *N Engl J Med.*, 1998, 339, 659-666.

[181] Ashihara, T; Haraguchi, R; Nakazawa, K; et al. The role of fibroblasts in complex fractionated electrograms during persistent/permanent atrial fibrillation: implications for electrogram-based catheter ablation. *Circ Res*, 2012, 110, 275-284.

[182] Aguilar, M; Qi, XY; Huang, H; Comtois, P; Nattel, S. Fibroblast electrical remodeling in heart failure and potential effects on atrial fibrillation. *Biophys J*, 2014, 107, 2444-2455.

[183] Burstein, B; Comtois, P; Michael, G; et al. Changes in connexin expression and the atrial fibrillation substrate in congestive heart failure. *Circ Res*, 2009, 105, 1213-1222.

[184] Nattel, S; Burstein, B; Dobrev, D. Atrial remodeling and atrial fibrillation: mechanisms and implications. *Circ Arrhythm Electrophysiol*, 2008, 1, 62-73.

[185] Nattel, S. Molecular and Cellular Mechanisms of Atrial Fibrosis in Atrial Fibrillation. *J Am Coll Cardiol EP*, 2017, 3, 425-435.

[186] McDowell, KS; Vadakkumpadan, F; Blake, R; et al. Mechanistic inquiry into the role of tissue remodeling in fibrotic lesions in human atrial fibrillation. *Biophys J*, 2013, 104, 2764-2773.

[187] Vasquez, C; Mohandas, P; Louie, KL; Benamer, N; Bapat, AC; Morley, GE. Enhanced fibroblast-myocyte interactions in response to cardiac injury. *Circ Res*, 2010, 107, 1011–20.

[188] Thery, C; Cosselin, B; Lekieffre, J; et al. Pathology of sinoatrial node. Correlations with electrocardiographic findings in 111 patients. *Am Heart I*, 1977, 93, 735-740.

[189] Spach, MS; Dolher, PC. Relating extracellular potentials and their derivatives to anisotropic propagation at a microscopic level in human cardiac muscle. *Circ Res*, 1986, 58, 356-371.

[190] Centurion, OA; Fukatani, M; Konoe, A; et al. Electrophysiological abnormalities of the atrial muscle in patients with sinus node dysfunction without tachyarrhythmias. *Int J Cardiol*, 1992, 37, 41-191.

[191] Centurión, OA; Isomoto, S; Fukatani, M; Shimizu, A; Hirata, T; Hano, O; Konoe, A; Tanigawa, M; Kaibara, M; Sakamoto, R; Yano, K. Relationship between atrial conduction defects and fractionated atrial endocardial electrograms in patients with sick sinus syndrome. *PACE*, 1993, 16, 2022-2033.

[192] Leier, CV; Meacham, JA; Schaal, SF. Prolonged atrial conduction: A major predisposing factor for the development of atriai flutter, *Circulation*, 1978, 57, 213-216.

[193] Mary-Rabine, L; Albert, A; Hordof, A; et al. The relationship of human atrial cellular electrophysiology to clinical function and uitrastrnctnre. *Circ Res*, 1983, 52, 188-199.

[194] Spach, MS. Miller, WT; Dolber, PC; et al. The functional role of structural complexities in the propagation of depolarization in the atrium of the dog. Cardiac conduction disturbances due to discontinuities of effective axial resistivity. *Circ Res*, 1982, 50, 175-191.

[195] Boineau, JP; Schuessler, RB. Mooney, CR; et al. Natural and evoked atrial flutter due to circus movement in dogs. *Am I Cardiol*, 1980, 45, 1167-1181.

[196] Boyden, PA; Tilley, LP; Albala, A; et al. Mechanism for atrial arrhythmias associated with cardiomyopathy: A study of feline hearts with primary myocardial disease. *Circulation*, 1984, 69, 1036-1047.

[197] Hatem, SN; Redheuil, A; Gandjbakhch, E. Cardiac adipose tissue and atrial fibrillation: the perils of adiposity. *Cardiovasc Res.*, 2016, 109, 502-509. https://doi.org/10.1093/cvr/cvw001 PMID: 26790475.

[198] Bouazizi, K; Rahhal, A; Kusmia, S; Evin, M; Defrance, C; Cluzel, P; et al. (2018) Differentiation and quantification of fibrosis, fat and fatty fibrosis in human left atrial myocardium using *ex vivo* MRI. *PLoS ONE*, 2018, 13(10), e0205104. https://doi.org/10.1371/journal.pone.0205104.

[199] Huber, A; Lamy, J; Rahhal, A; Evin, M; Atassi, F; Defrance, C; et al. Cardiac MR Strain: A Noninvasive Biomarker of Fibrofatty Remodeling of the Left Atrial Myocardium. *Radiology.*, 2018, 286.

[200] Ferreira, VM; Piechnik, SK; Robson, MD; Neubauer, S; Karamitsos, TD. Myocardial tissue characterization by magnetic resonance imaging: novel applications of T1 and T2 mapping. *J Thorac Imaging.*, 2014, 29, 147-154. https://doi.org/10.1097/RTI.0000000000000077 PMID, 24576837.

[201] Mewton, N; Liu, CY; Croisille, P; Bluemke, D; Lima, J. Assessment of Myocardial Fibrosis with Cardiac Magnetic Resonance. *J Am Coll Cardiol.*, 2011, 57, 891-903. https://doi.org/10.1016/j.jacc.2010.11.013. PMID: 21329834.

[202] Bohnen, S; Radunski, UK; Lund, GK; Ojeda, F; Looft, Y; Senel, M; et al. Tissue characterization by T1 and T2 mapping cardiovascular magnetic resonance imaging to monitor myocardial inflammation in healing myocarditis. *Eur Heart J Cardiovasc Imaging.*, 2017, 744-751.

[203] Puntmann, VO; Voigt, T; Chen, Z; Mayr, M; Karim, R; Rhode, K; et al. Native T1 Mapping in Differentiation of Normal Myocardium From Diffuse Disease in Hypertrophic and Dilated Cardiomyopathy.

J Am Coll Cardiol Cardiovasc Imaging., 2013, 6, 475-484. https://doi.org/10.1016/j.jcmg.2012.08.019. PMID: 23498674.

[204] Messroghli, DR; Walters, K; Plein, S; Sparrow, P; Friedrich, MG; Ridgway, JP; et al. Myocardial T1 mapping: Application to patients with acute and chronic myocardial infarction. *Magn Reson Med.*, 2007, 58, 34-40. https://doi.org/10.1002/mrm.21272. PMID: 1765962 2.

[205] Dass, S; Suttie, J; Piechnik, S; Ferreira, V; Holloway, C; Banerjee, R; et al. Myocardial Tissue Characterization Using Magnetic Resonance Non-contrast T1 Mapping in Hypertrophic and Dilated Cardiomyopathy. *Circ Cardiovasc Imaging.*, 2012, 5, 726-733.

[206] Kellman, P; Hansen, MS. T1-mapping in the heart: accuracy and precision. *J Cardiovasc Magn Reson.*, 2014, 16, 1-20. https://doi.org/10.1186/1532-429X-16-1.

[207] Beinart, R; Khurram, IM; Liu, S; Yarmohammadi, H; Halperin, HR; Bluemke, DA; et al. Cardiac magnetic resonance T1 mapping of left atrial myocardium. *Heart Rhythm.*, 2013, 10, 1325-1331. https://doi.org/10.1016/j.hrthm.2013.05.003. PMID, 23643513.

[208] Hamilton-Craig, CR; Strudwick, MW; Galloway, GJ. T1 Mapping for Myocardial Fibrosis by Cardiac Magnetic Resonance RelaxometryÐA Comprehensive Technical Review. *Front Cardiovasc Med.*, 2017, 3, 1-11.

[209] Germain, P; El Ghannudi, S; Mi-Young, J; Ohlmann, P; Epailly, E; Roy, C; et al. Clinical Medicine Insights: Cardiology. *Lib Acad.*, 2014, 8, 1-11.

[210] Hordof, AJ; Edie, R; Malm, JR; et al. Electrophysiologic properties and response to pharmacologic agents of fibers from diseased human atria. *Circulation*, 1976, 54, 774-779.

[211] Josephson, ME; Kastor, IA; Morganroth, I. Electrocardiographic left atrial enlargement: Electrophysiologic, echocardiographic and hemodynamic correlates. *Am I Cardiol*, 1977, 39, 967-971.

[212] Mazzoleni, A; Wolff, R; Wolff, L; et al. Correlation between component cardiac weights and electrocardiographic patterns in 185 cases. *Circulation*, 1964, 30, 808-829.

[213] Ross, C. Effect of hypertension on the P wave of the ECC. *Br Heart*, 11963, 25, 460-464.

[214] Simpson, RUr; Amaral. Foster IR. et al., Thresholds, refractory periods, and conduction times of normal and diseased human atrium. *Am Heart*, 1988, 116, 1080-1090.

[215] Killip, T; Cault, IH. Mode of onset of atrial fihrillation in man. *Am Heart I*, 1965, 70, 172-179.

[216] Li, D; Shinagawa, K; Pang, L; et al. Effects of angiotensin-converting enzyme inhibition on the development of the atrial fibrillation substrate in dogs with ventricular tachypacing-induced congestive heart failure. *Circulation*, 2001, 104, 2608-2614.

[217] Burstein, B; Nattel, S. Atrial structural remodeling as an antiarrhythmic target. *J Cardiovasc Pharmacol*, 2008, 52, 4-10.

[218] Chen, Y; Surinkaew, S; Wu, CT; et al. JAK-STAT signalling and the atrial fibrillation-promoting fibrotic substrate: pathogenic role and possible therapeutic target. *Cardiovasc Res*, 2017, 113, 310-320.

[219] Cardin, S; Guasch, E; Luo, X; et al. Role for MicroRNA-21 in atrial profibrillatory fibrotic remodeling associated with experimental postinfarction heart failure. *Circ Arrhythm Electrophysiol*, 2012, 5, 1027-1035.

[220] Huang, Z; Chen, XJ; Qian, C; et al. Signal transducer and activator of transcription 3/microRNA-21 feedback loop contributes to atrial fibrillation by promoting atrial fibrosis in a rat sterile pericarditis model. *Circ Arrhythm Electrophysiol*, 2016, 9, e003396.

[221] He, X; Zhang, K; Gao, X; et al. Rapid atrial pacing induces myocardial fibrosis by down-regulating Smad7 via microRNA-21 in rabbit. *Heart Vessels*, 2016, 31, 1696-708.

[222] Harada, M; Luo, X; Qi, XY; et al. Transient receptor potential canonical-3 channel-dependent fibroblast regulation in atrial fibrillation. *Circulation*, 2012, 126, 2051-2064.

[223] Shimano, M; Tsuji, Y; Inden, Y; et al. Pioglitazone a peroxisome proliferator-activated receptor- gamma activator, attenuates atrial fibrosis and atrial fibrillation promotion in rabbits with congestive heart failure. *Heart Rhythm*, 2008, 5, 451-459.

[224] Savelieva, I; Kakouros, N; Kourliouros, A; Camm, AJ. Upstream therapies for management of atrial fibrillation: review of clinical evidence and implications for European Society of Cardiology guidelines. Part I: primary prevention. *Europace*, 2011, 13, 308-328.

[225] Goldman, MR; Brady, TJ; Pykett, IL; et al. Quantification of experimental myocardial infarction using nuclear magnetic resonance imaging and paramagnetic ion contrast enhancement in excised canine hearts. *Circulation*, 1982, 66, 1012-1016.

[226] Han, FT; Akoum, N; Marrouche, N. Value of magnetic resonance imaging in guiding atrial fibrillation management. *Can J Cardiol*, 2013, 29, 1194-1202.

[227] Kim, RJ; Fieno, DS; Parrish, TB; et al. Relationship of MRI delayed contrast enhancement to irreversible injury, infarct age, and contractile function. *Circulation*, 1999, 100, 1992-2002.

[228] Weinmann, HJ; Brasch, RC; Press, WR; Wesbey, GE. Characteristics of gadolinium-DTPA complex: a potential NMR contrast agent. *Am J Roentgenol*, 1984, 142, 619-624.

[229] Gal, P; Marrouche, NF. Magnetic resonance imaging of atrial fibrosis: redefining atrial fibrillation to a syndrome. *Eur Heart J*, 2017, 38, 14-19.

[230] Allessie, M; Ausma, J; Schotten, U. Electrical, contractile and structural remodeling during atrial fibrillation. *Cardiovasc Res*, 2002, 54, 230-246.

[231] Burstein, B; Nattel, S. Atrial fibrosis: mechanisms and clinical relevance in atrial fibrillation. *J Am Coll Cardiol*, 2008, 51, 802-809.

[232] Kim, RJ; Chen, EL; Lima, JA; Judd, RM. Myocardial Gd-DTPA kinetics determine MRI contrast enhancement and reflect the extent and severity of myocardial injury after acute reperfused infarction. *Circulation*, 1996, 94, 3318-3326.

[233] Marrouche, NF; Wilber, D; Hindricks, G; et al. Association of atrial tissue fibrosis identified by delayed enhancement MRI and atrial fibrillation catheter ablation: the DECAAF study. *JAMA*, 2014, 311, 498-506.

[234] Yerram, P; Saab, G; Karuparthi, PR; Hayden, MR; Khanna, R. Nephrogenic systemic fibrosis: a mysterious disease in patients with renal failure–role of gadolinium-based contrast media in causation and the beneficial effect of intravenous sodium thiosulfate. *Clin J Am Soc Nephrol*, 2007, 2, 258-263.

[235] Akoum, N; McGann, C; Vergara, G; et al. Atrial fibrosis quantified using late gadolinium enhancement MRI is associated with sinus node dysfunction requiring pacemaker implant. *J Cardiovasc Electrophysiol*, 2012, 23, 44-50.

[236] Allessie, M; Ausma, J; Schotten, U. Electrical, contractile and structural remodeling during atrial fibrillation. *Cardiovasc Res*, 2002, 54(2), 230-246.

[237] Kourliouros, A; Savelieva, I; Kiotsekoglou, A; et al. Current concepts in the pathogenesis of atrial fibrillation. *Am Heart J*, 2009, 157(2), 243-52.

[238] Scharf, C; Sneider, M; Case, I; et al. Anatomy of the pulmonary veins in patients with atrial fibrillation and effects of segmental ostial ablation analyzed by computed tomography. *J Cardiovasc Electrophysiol*, 2003, 14(2), 150 -155.

[239] Cronin, P; Sneider, MB; Kazerooni, EA; et al. MDCT of the Left Atrium and Pulmonary Veins in Planning Radiofrequency Ablation for Atrial Fibrillation: A How-To Guide. *AJR Am J Roentgenol*, 2004, 183(3), 767-778.

[240] Tsao, HM; WU, MH; Yu, WC; et al. Role of right middle pulmonary vein in patients with paroxysmal atrial fibrillation. *J Cardiovasc Electrophysiol*, 2001, 12(12), 1353 -1357.

[241] Marom, EM; Herndon, JE; Kim, YH; et al. Variations in pulmonary venous drainage to the left atrium: implications for radiofrequency ablation. *Radiology*, 2004, 230(3), 824-829.

[242] Ho, SY; Cabrera, JA; Sánchez-Quintana, D. Anatomy of the pulmonary vein-atrium junction. In: Chen SA, Haïssaguerre M, Zipes DP, Eds. *Thoracic vein arrhythmias. Mechanisms and treatment.* Oxford: Blackwell Futura, 2004, pp. 42-53.

[243] Oral, H; Pappone, C; Chugh, A; et al. Circumferential pulmonary vein ablation for chronic atrial fibrillation. *N Engl J Med*, 2006, 354(9), 934-941.

[244] Fisher, JD; Spinelli, MA; Mookherjee, D; Krumerman, AK; Palma, EC. Atrial fibrillation ablation: reaching the mainstream. Pacing Clin *Electrophysiol*, 2006, 29(5), 523-537.

[245] Lim, KT; Matsuo, S; O'Neill, MD; et al. Catheter ablation of persistent and permanent atrial fibrillation: Bordeaux experience. *Expert Rev Cardiovasc Ther*, 2007, 5(4), 655-662.

[246] Oral, H; Scharf, C; Chugh, A; et al. Catheter ablation for paroxysmal atrial fibrillation. *Circulation.*, 2003, 108, 2355-2360.

[247] Oakes, RS; Badger, TJ; Kholmovski, EG; et al. Detection and quantification of left atrial structural remodeling with delayed-enhancement magnetic resonance imaging in patients with atrial fibrillation. *Circulation.*, 2009, 119, 1758-1767.

[248] Akoum, N; Daccarett, M; McGann, C; et al. Atrial fibrosis helps select the appropriate patient and strategy in catheter ablation of atrial fibrillation: a DE-MRI guided approach. *J Cardiovasc Electrophysiol.*, 2011, 22(1), 16-22.

[249] McGann, CJ; Kholmovski, EG; Oakes, RS; et al. New magnetic resonance imaging-based method for defining the extent of left atrial wall injury after the ablation of atrial fibrillation. *J Am Coll Cardiol.*, 2008, 52, 1263-1271.

[250] Peters, DC; Wylie, JV; Hauser, TH; et al. Detection of pulmonary vein and left atrial scar after catheter ablation with three-dimensional navigator-gated delayed enhancement MR imaging: initial experience1. *Radiology.*, 2007, 243, 690-695.

[251] Harrison, JL; Jensen, HK; Peel, SA; et al. Cardiac magnetic resonance and electroanatomical mapping of acute and chronic atrial ablation injury: a histological validation study. *Eur Heart J*, 2014, 35, 1486-1495.

[252] Chrispin, J; Ipek, EG; Habibi, M; et al. Clinical predictors of cardiac magnetic resonance late gadolinium enhancement in patients with atrial fibrillation. *Europace*, 2017, 19, 371-377.

[253] Akoum, N; Fernandez, G; Wilson, B; McGann, C; Kholmovski, E; Marrouche, N. Association of atrial fibrosis quantified using LGE-MRI with atrial appendage thrombus and spontaneous contrast on transesophageal echocardiography in patients with atrial fibrillation. *J Cardiovasc Electr*, 2013, 24, 1104-1109.

[254] Cochet, H; Mouries, A; Nivet, H; et al. Age, atrial fibrillation, and structural heart disease are the main determinants of left atrial fibrosis detected by delayed-enhanced magnetic resonance imaging in a general cardiology population. *J Cardiovasc Electrophysiol*, 2015, 26, 484-492.

[255] McGann, C; Akoum, N; Patel, A; et al. Atrial fibrillation ablation outcome is predicted by left atrial remodeling on MRI. *Circ Arrhythm Electrophysiol*, 2014, 7, 23-30.

[256] Malcolme-Lawes, LC; Juli, C; Karim, R; et al. Automated analysis of atrial late gadolinium enhancement imaging that correlates with endocardial voltage and clinical outcomes: a 2-center study. *Heart Rhythm*, 2013, 10, 1184-1191.

[257] Khurram, IM; Beinart, R; Zipunnikov, V; et al. Magnetic resonance image intensity ratio, a normalized measure to enable interpatient comparability of left atrial fibrosis. *Heart Rhythm*, 2014, 11, 85-92.

[258] Fukumoto, K; Habibi, M; Gucuk Ipek, E; et al. Comparison of preexisting and ablation-induced late gadolinium enhancement on left atrial magnetic resonance imaging. *Heart Rhythm*, 2015, 12, 668-672.

[259] Bisbal, F; Guiu, E; Cabanas-Grandio, P; et al. CMR-guided approach to localize and ablate gaps in repeat AF ablation procedure. *J Am Coll Cardiol Img*, 2014, 7, 653-663.

[260] Harrison, JL; Sohns, C; Linton, NW; et al. Repeat left atrial catheter ablation: cardiac magnetic resonance prediction of endocardial voltage and gaps in ablation lesion sets. *Circ Arrhythm Electrophysiol*, 2015, 8, 270-278.

[261] Benito, EM; Carlosena-Remirez, A; Guasch, E; et al. Left atrial fibrosis quantification by late gadolinium-enhanced magnetic resonance: a new method to standardize the thresholds for reproducibility. *Europace*, 2017, 19(8), 1272-1279.

[262] Kawel, N; Turkbey, EB; Carr, JJ; et al. Normal left ventricular myocardial thickness for middle-aged and older subjects with steady-state free precession cardiac magnetic resonance: the multi-Ethnic Study of Atherosclerosis. *Circ Cardiovasc Imaging*, 2012, 5, 500-508.

[263] Appelbaum, E; Manning, WJ. Left atrial fibrosis by late gadolinium enhancement cardiovascular magnetic resonance predicts recurrence of atrial fibrillation after pulmonary vein isolation: do you see what I see? *Circ Arrhythm Electrophysiol*, 2014, 7, 2-4.

[264] Bois, JP; Glockner, J; Young, PM; et al. Low incidence of left atrial delayed enhancement with MRI in patients with AF: a single-centre experience. *Open Heart*, 2017, 4, e000546.

[265] Chia, JM; Fischer, SE; Wickline, SA; Lorenz, CH. Performance of QRS detection for cardiac magnetic resonance imaging with a novel vector cardiographic triggering method. *J Magn Reson Imaging*, 2000, 12, 678-688.

[266] Beinart, R; Nazarian, S. Role of magnetic resonance imaging in atrial fibrillation ablation. *Curr Treat Options Cardiovasc Med*, 2014, 16, 316.

[267] Siebermair, J; Kholmovski, EG; Marrouche, NF. Assessment of left atrial fibrosis by late gadolinium enhancement magnetic resonance imaging: Methodology and clinical implications. *JACC Clin Electrophysiol*, 2017, 3(8), 791-802.

[268] Vijayakumar, S; Kholmovski, EG; Haslam, MM; Burgon, NS; Marrouche, NF. Dependence of image quality of late gadolinium enhancement MRI of left atrium on number of patients imaged: results of multi-center trial DECAAF. *J Cardiovasc Magn Reson*, 2014, 16, 146.

[269] Higuchi, K; Cates, J; Gardner, G; Morris, A; Burgon, N; Akoum, N; Marrouche, NF. The spatial distribution of late gadolinium enhancement of left atrial magnetic resonance imaging in patients with atrial fibrillation. *J Am Coll Cardiol EP*, 2018, 4, 49-58.

[270] Platonov, PG; Mitrofanova, LB; Orshanskaya, V; Ho, SY. Structural abnormalities in atrial walls are associated with presence and

persistency of atrial fibrillation but not with age. *J Am Coll Cardiol*, 2011, 58, 2225-2232.

[271] Tanaka, K; Zlochiver, S; Vikstrom, KL; et al. Spatial distribution of fibrosis governs fibrillation wave dynamics in the posterior left atrium during heart failure. *Circ Res*, 2007, 101, 839-847.

[272] Corradi, D; Callegari, S; Benussi, S; et al. Myocyte changes and their left atrial distribution in patients with chronic atrial fibrillation related to mitral valve disease. *Hum Pathol*, 2005, 36, 1080-1089.

[273] Asirvatham, SJ; Gard, JJ. Wrinkles in the atrium: age, atrial fibrillation, or something else. *J Am Coll Cardiol*, 2011, 58, 2233-2235.

[274] Hori, Y; Nakahara, S; Tsukada, N; et al. The influence of the external structures in atrial fibrillation patients: relationship to focal low voltage areas in the left atrium. *Int J Cardiol*, 2015, 181, 225-231.

[275] Lachman, N; Syed, FF; Habib, A; et al. Correlative anatomy for the electrophysiologist, Part I: the pericardial space, oblique sinus, transverse sinus. *J Cardiovasc Electrophysiol*, 2010, 21, 1421-1426.

[276] Hunter, RJ; Liu, Y; Lu, Y; Wang, W; Schilling, RJ. Left atrial wall stress distribution and its relationship to electrophysiologic remodeling in persistent atrial fibrillation. *Circ Arrhythm Electrophysiol*, 2012, 5, 351-360.

[277] Nakahara, S; Yamaguchi, T; Hori, Y; et al. Spatial relation between left atrial anatomical contact areas and circular activation in persistent atrial fibrillation. *J Cardiovasc Electrophysiol*, 2016, 27, 515-523.

[278] Verma, A; Jiang, CY; Betts, TR; et al. Approaches to catheter ablation for persistent atrial fibrillation. *N Engl J Med*, 2015, 372, 1812-1822.

[279] Yang, G; Zhuang, X; Khan, H; Haldar, S; Nyktari, E; Li, L; et al. Fully automatic segmentation and objective assessment of atrial scars for long-standing persistent atrial fibrillation patients using late gadolinium-enhanced MRI. *Med. Phys.*, 2018, 45 (4), 1562-1576.

[280] Akoum, N; Daccarett, M; McGann, C; et al. Atrial fibrosis helps select the appropriate patient and strategy in catheter ablation of atrial fibrillation: a DE-MRI guided approach. *J Cardiovasc Electrophysiol*, 2011, 22, 16-22.

[281] Marrouche, NF; Wilber, D; Hindricks, G; et al. Association of atrial tissue fibrosis identified by delayed enhancement MRI and atrial fibrillation catheter ablation: the DECAAF study. *JAMA*, 2014, 311, 498-506.

[282] McGann, C; Akoum, N; Patel, A; et al. Atrial fibrillation ablation outcome is predicted by left atrial remodeling on MRI. *Circ Arrhythm Electrophysiol*, 2014, 7, 23-30.

[283] Rolf, S; Kircher, S; Arya, A; et al. Tailored atrial substrate modification based on low-voltage areas in catheter ablation of atrial fibrillation. *Circ Arrhythm Electrophysiol*, 2014, 7, 825-833.

[284] Yang, G; Yang, B; Wei, Y; et al. Catheter ablation of nonparoxysmal atrial fibrillation using electrophysiologically guided substrate modification during sinus rhythm after pulmonary vein isolation. *Circ Arrhythm Electrophysiol*, 2016, 9, e 003382.

[285] Yamaguchi, T; Tsuchiya, T; Nakahara, S; et al. Efficacy of left atrial voltage-based catheter ablation of persistent atrial fibrillation. *J Cardiovasc Electrophysiol*, 2016, 27, 1055-1063.

[286] Jadidi, AS; Lehrmann, H; Keyl, C; et al. Ablation of persistent atrial fibrillation targeting low-voltage areas with selective activation characteristics. *Circ Arrhythm Electrophysiol*, 2016, 9, e002962.

[287] Ramanathan, C; Ghanem, RN; Jia, P; et al. Noninvasive electrocardiographic imaging for cardiac electrophysiology and arrhythmia. *Nat Med*, 2004, 10, 422-428.

[288] Oster, HS; Taccardi, B; Lux, RL; et al. Noninvasive electrocardiographic imaging: reconstruction of epicardial potentials, electrograms, and isochrones and localization of single and multiple electrocardiac events. *Circulation*, 1997, 96, 1012-1024.

[289] Burnes, JE; Taccardi, B; Rudy, Y. A noninvasive imaging modality for cardiac arrhythmias. *Circulation*, 2000, 102, 2152-2158.

[290] Wang, Y; Cuculich, PS; Zhang, J; et al. Noninvasive electroanatomic mapping of human ventricular arrhythmias with electrocardiographic imaging. *Sci Transl Med*, 2011, 3, 98-104.

[291] Haïssaguerre, M; Hocini, M; Shah, AJ; et al. Noninvasive panoramic mapping of human atrial fibrillation mechanisms: a feasibility report. *J Cardiovasc Electrophysiol*, 2013, 24, 711-717.

[292] Shah, AJ; Hocini, M; Xhaet, O; et al. Validation of novel 3D electrocardiographic mapping of atrial tachycardias by invasive mapping and ablation: a multicenter study. *J AmColl Cardiol*, 2013, 62, 889-897.

[293] Ploux, S; Lumens, J; Whinnett, Z; et al. Noninvasive electrocardiographic mapping to improve patient selection for cardiac resynchronization therapy: beyond QRS duration and left bundle branch block morphology. *J Am Coll Cardiol*, 2013, 61, 2435-2443.

[294] Narayan, SM; Krummen, DE; Shivkumar, K; et al. Treatment of atrial fibrillation by the ablation of localized sources: CONFIRM (Conventional Ablation for Atrial Fibrillation With or Without Focal Impulse and Rotor Modulation) trial. *J Am Coll Cardiol*, 2012, 60, 628-636.

[295] Haïssaguerre, M; Hocini, M; Denis, A; et al. Driver domains in persistent atrial fibrillation. *Circulation*, 2014, 130, 530-538.

[296] Kostin, S; Klein, G; Szalay, Z; et al. Structural correlate of atrial fibrillation in human patients. *Cardiovasc Res*, 2002, 54, 361-379.

[297] Platonov, PG; Mitrofanova, LB; Orshanskaya, V; et al. Structural abnormalities in atrial walls are associated with presence and persistency of atrial fibrillation but not with age. *J Am Coll Cardiol*, 2011, 58, 2225-2232.

[298] Burstein, B; Nattel, S. Atrial fibrosis: mechanisms and clinical relevance in atrial fibrillation. *J Am Coll Cardiol*, 2008, 51, 802-809.

[299] Zlochiver, S; Muñoz, V; Vikstrom, KL; et al. Electrotonic myofibroblast-to-myocyte coupling increases propensity to reentrant arrhythmias in two-dimensional cardiac monolayers. *Biophys J*, 2008, 95, 4469-4480.

[300] Everett, TH; 4th, Wilson, EE; Verheule, S; et al. Structural atrial remodeling alters the substrate and spatiotemporal organization of atrial fibrillation: a comparison in canine models of structural and

electrical atrial remodeling. *Am J Physiol Heart Circ Physiol*, 2006, 291, H2911-H2923.

[301] Tanaka, K; Zlochiver, S; Vikstrom, KL; et al. Spatial distribution of fibrosis governs fibrillation wave dynamics in the posterior left atrium during heart failure. *Circ Res*, 2007, 101, 839-847.

[302] Oakes, RS; Badger, TJ; Kholmovski, EG; et al. Detection and quantification of left atrial structural remodeling using delayed enhancement MRI in patients with atrial fibrillation. *Circulation*, 2009, 119, 1758-1767.

[303] McGann, C; Akoum, N; Patel, A; et al. Atrial fibrillation ablation outcome is predicted by left atrial remodeling on MRI. *Circ Arrhythm Electrophysiol*, 2014, 7, 23-30.

[304] Cochet, H; Dubois, R; Yamashita, S; Al Jefairi, N; Berte, B; Sellal, JM; et al. Relationship between fibrosis detected on late gadolinium-enhanced cardiac magnetic resonance and reentrant activity assessed with electrocardiographic imaging in human persistent atrial fibrillation. *J Am Coll Cardiol EP*, 2018, 4(1), 17-29.

[305] Li, D; Zhang, L; Kneller, J; Nattel, S. Potential ionic mechanism for repolarization differences between canine right and left atrium. *Circ Res*, 2001, 88, 1168-1175.

[306] Jadidi, AS; Cochet, H; Shah, AJ; et al. Inverse relationship between fractionated electrograms and atrial fibrosis in persistent atrial fibrillation: combined magnetic resonance imaging and high-density mapping. *J Am Coll Cardiol*, 2013, 62, 802-812.

[307] Chrispin, J; Gucuk Ipek, E; Zahid, S; et al. Lack of regional association between atrial late gadolinium enhancement on cardiac magnetic resonance and atrial fibrillation rotors. *Heart Rhythm*, 2016, 13, 654-660.

[308] Gonzales, MJ; Vincent, KP; Rappel, WJ; et al. Structural contributions to fibrillatory rotors in a patient-derived computational model of the atria. *Europace*, 2014, 16 Suppl 4, iv3–10.

[309] Hansen, BJ; Zhao, J; Csepe, TA; et al. Atrial fibrillation driven by micro-anatomic intramural reentry revealed by simultaneous sub-

epicardial and sub-endocardial optical mapping in explanted human hearts. *Eur Heart J*, 2015, 36, 2390-2401.

[310] Zahid, S; Cochet, H; Boyle, PM; et al. Patient derived models link re-entrant driver localization in atrial fibrillation to fibrosis spatial pattern. *Cardiovasc Res*, 2016, 110, 443-454.

[311] Kottkamp, H; Schreiber, D; Moser, F; Rieger, A. Therapeutic approaches to atrial fibrillation ablation targeting atrial fibrosis. *J Am Coll Cardiol EP*, 2017, 3, 643-653.

[312] Kottkamp, H; Berg, J; Bender, R; Rieger, A; Schreiber, D. Box isolation of fibrotic areas (BIFA): a patient-tailored substrate modification approach for ablation of atrial fibrillation. *J Cardiovasc Electrophysiol*, 2016, 27, 22-30.

[313] Schreiber, D; Rieger, A; Moser, F; Kottkamp, H. Catheter ablation of atrial fibrillation with box isolation of fibrotic areas: lessons of fibrosis distribution and extent, clinical characteristics and their impact on long-term outcome. *J Cardiovasc Electrophysiol*, 2017, 28(9), 971-983.

[314] Mahnkopf, C; Badger, TJ; Burgon, NS; et al. Evaluation of the left atrial substrate in patients with lone atrial fibrillation using delayed-enhanced MRI: implications for disease progression and response to catheter ablation. *Heart Rhythm*, 2010, 7, 1475-1481.

[315] Kottkamp, H; Schreiber, D. The substrate in "early persistent" atrial fibrillation: Arrhythmia induced, risk factor induced, or from a specific fibrotic atrial cardiomyopathy? *J Am Coll Cardiol EP*, 2016, 2, 140-142.

[316] Stiles, MK; John, B; Wong, CX; et al. Paroxysmal lone atrial fibrillation is associated with an abnormal atrial substrate: characterizing the "second factor." *J Am Coll Cardiol*, 2009, 53, 1182-1191.

[317] Kottkamp, H; Bender, R; Berg, J. Catheter ablation of atrial fibrillation: how to modify the substrate? *J Am Coll Cardiol*, 2015, 65, 196-206.

[318] Verma, A; Wazni, OM; Marrouche, NF; et al. Preexistent left atrial scarring in patients undergoing pulmonary vein antrum isolation: an

independent predictor of procedural failure. *J Am Coll Cardiol*, 2005, 45, 285-292.

[319] Kapa, S; Desjardins, B; Callans, DJ; Marchlinski, FE; Dixit, S. Contact electroanatomic mapping derived voltage criteria for characterizing left atrial scar in patients undergoing ablation for atrial fibrillation. *J Cardiovasc Electrophysiol*, 2014, 25, 1044-1052.

[320] Rolf, S; Kircher, S; Arya, A; et al. Tailored atrial substrate modification based on low-voltage areas in catheter ablation of atrial fibrillation. *Circ Arrhythm Electrophysiol*, 2014, 7, 825-833.

[321] Yang, G; Yang, B; Wei, Y; et al. Catheter ablation of non-paroxysmal atrial fibrillation using electrophysiologically guided substrate modification during sinus rhythm after pulmonary vein isolation. *Circ Arrhythm Electrophysiol*, 2016, 9, e003382.

[322] Anter, E; Tschabrunn, CM; Josephson, ME. High-resolution mapping of scar-related atrial arrhythmias using smaller electrodes with closer interelectrode spacing. *Circ Arrhythm Electrophysiol*, 2015, 8, 537-545.

[323] Yagishita, A; De Oliveira, S; Cakulev, I; et al. Correlation of left atrial voltage distribution between sinus rhythm and atrial fibrillation: identifying structural remodeling by 3-D electroanatomic mapping irrespective of the rhythm. *J Cardiovasc Electrophysiol*, 2016, 27, 905-912.

[324] Yagishita, A; Sparano, D; Cakulev, I; et al. Identification and electrophysiological characterization of early left atrial structural remodeling as a predictor for atrial fibrillation recurrence after pulmonary vein isolation. *J Cardiovasc Electrophysiol*, 2017, 28, 642-650.

[325] Kuck, KH; Hoffmann, BA; Ernst, S; et al., for the Gap-AF-AFNET 1 Investigators. Impact of complete versus incomplete circumferential lines around the pulmonary veins during catheter ablation of paroxysmal atrial fibrillation: results from the Gap–Atrial Fibrillation–German Atrial Fibrillation Competence Network 1 Trial. *Circ Arrhythm Electrophysiol*, 2016, 9, e003337.

[326] Yagishita, A; Gimbel, JR; De Oliveira, S; et al. Long-term outcome of left atrial voltage-guided substrate ablation during atrial fibrillation: a novel adjunctive ablation strategy. *J Cardiovasc Electrophysiol*, 2017, 28, 147-155.

[327] Kumagai, K; Muraoka, S; Mitsutake, C; Takashima, H; Nakashima, H. A new approach for complete isolation of the posterior left atrium including pulmonary veins for atrial fibrillation. *J Cardiovasc Electrophysiol*, 2007, 18, 1047-1052.

[328] Yamaguchi, T; Tsuchiya, T; Nakahara, S; et al. Efficacy of left atrial voltage-based catheter ablation of persistent atrial fibrillation. *J Cardiovasc Electrophysiol*, 2016, 27, 1055-1063.

[329] Jadidi, AS; Lehrmann, H; Keyl, C; et al. Ablation of persistent atrial fibrillation targeting low-voltage areas with selective activation characteristics. *Circ Arrhythm Electrophysiol*, 2016, 9. pii: e002962.

[330] Narayan, SM; Krummen, DE; Shivkumar, K; Clopton, P; Rappel, WJ; Miller, JM. Treatment of atrial fibrillation by the ablation of localized sources: CONFIRM (Conventional Ablation for Atrial Fibrillation With or Without Focal Impulse and Rotor Modulation) trial. *J Am Coll Cardiol*, 2012, 60, 628–36.

[331] Haissaguerre, M; Hocini, M; Denis, A; et al. Driver domains in persistent atrial fibrillation. *Circulation*, 2014, 130, 530-538.

[332] McGann, C; Akoum, N; Patel, A; et al. Atrial fibrillation ablation outcome is predicted by left atrial remodelling on MRI. *Circ Arrhythm Electrophysiol*, 2014, 7, 23-30.

[333] Jadidi, A; Müller-Edenborn, B; Chen, J; Keyl, C; Weber, R; Allgeier, J; et al. The duration of the amplified sinus-P-wave identifies presence of left atrial low voltage substrate and predicts outcome after pulmonary vein isolation in patients with persistent atrial fibrillation. *J Am Coll Cardiol EP*, 2018, 4, 531-543.

[334] Bayes de Luna, A; Fort de Ribot, R; Trilla, E; et al. Electrocardiographic and vectorcardiographic study of interatrial conduction disturbances with left atrial retrograde activation. *J Electrocardiol*, 1985, 18, 1-13.

[335] Surawicz, B. Chou's Electrocardiography in Clinical Practice. New York, NY: Elsevier, 2008.

[336] Vincenti, A; Rota, M; Spinelli, M; et al. A noninvasive index of atrial remodeling in patients with paroxysmal and persistent atrial fibrillation: a pilot study. *J Electrocardiol*, 2012, 45, 109-115.

[337] Lin, Y; Yang, B; Garcia, FC; et al. Comparison of left atrial electrophysiologic abnormalities during sinus rhythm in patients with different type of atrial fibrillation. *J Interv Card Electrophysiol*, 2014, 39, 57-67.

[338] Platonov, PG. P-wave morphology: underlying mechanisms and clinical implications. *Annals Ann Noninvasive Electrocardiol*, 2012, 17, 161-169.

[339] Fukunami, M; Yamada, T; Ohmori, M; et al. Detection of patients at risk for paroxysmal atrial fibrillation during sinus rhythm by P wave triggered signal-averaged electrocardiogram. *Circulation*, 1991, 83, 162-169.

[340] Aytemir, K; Amasyali, B; Kose, S; et al. Maximum P-wave duration and P-wave dispersion predict recurrence of paroxysmal atrial fibrillation in patients with Wolff-Parkinson-White syndrome after successful radiofrequency catheter ablation. *J Interv Card Electrophysiol*, 2004, 11, 21-27.

[341] Blanche, C; Tran, N; Rigamonti, F; Burri, H; Zimmermann, M. Value of P-wave signal averaging to predict atrial fibrillation recurrences after pulmonary vein isolation. *Europace*, 2013, 15, 198-204.

[342] Caldwell, J; Koppikar, S; Barake, W; et al. Prolonged P-wave duration is associated with atrial fibrillation recurrence after successful pulmonary vein isolation for paroxysmal atrial fibrillation. *J Interv Card Electrophysiol*, 2014, 39, 131-138.

[343] Wu, JT; Long, DY; Dong, JZ; et al. Advanced interatrial block predicts clinical recurrence of atrial fibrillation after catheter ablation. *J Cardiol*, 2016, 68, 352-356.

[344] Mugnai, G; Chierchia, GB; De Asmundis, C; et al. P-wave indices as predictors of atrial fibrillation recurrence after pulmonary vein

isolation in normal left atrial size. *J Cardiovasc Med*, 2016, 17, 194-200.

[345] Wang, YS; Chen, GY; Li, XH; Zhou, X; Li, YG. Prolonged P-wave duration is associated with atrial fibrillation recurrence after radiofrequency catheter ablation: a systematic review and meta-analysis. *Int J Cardiol*, 2017, 227, 355-359.

[346] Ogawa, M; Kumagai, K; Vakulenko, M; et al. Reduction of P-wave duration and successful pulmonary vein isolation in patients with atrial fibrillation. *J Cardiovasc Electrophysiol*, 2007, 18, 931-938.

[347] Chalfoun, N; Harnick, D; Pe, E; Undavia, M; Mehta, D; Gomes, JA. Reverse electrical remodeling of the atria post cardioversion in patients who remain in sinus rhythm assessed by signal averaging of the P-wave. *Pacing Clin Electrophysiol*, 2007, 30, 502-509.

[348] Rivard, L; Hocini, M; Rostock, T; et al. Improved outcome following restoration of sinus rhythm prior to catheter ablation of persistent atrial fibrillation: a comparative multicenter study. *Heart Rhythm*, 2012, 9, 1025-1030.

[349] Haissaguerre, M; Hocini, M; Denis, A; et al. Driver domains in persistent atrial fibrillation. *Circulation*, 2014, 130, 530-538.

[350] Knecht, S; Sohal, M; Deisenhofer, I; et al. Multicentre evaluation of non-invasive biatrial mapping for persistent atrial fibrillation ablation: the AFACART study. *Europace*, 2017, 19, 1302-1309.

[351] Zhao, J; Hansen, BJ; Wang, Y; Csepe, TA; Sul, LV; Tang, A; et al. Three-dimensional Integrated Functional, Structural, and Computational Mapping to Define the Structural "Fingerprints" of Heart-Specific Atrial Fibrillation Drivers in Human Heart *Ex Vivo*. *J Am Heart Assoc.*, 2017, 6, e005922. DOI: 10.1161/JAHA.117.005922.

[352] McDowell, KS; Zahid, S; Vadakkumpadan, F; Blauer, J; MacLeod, RS; Trayanova, NA. Virtual Electrophysiological Study of Atrial Fibrillation in Fibrotic Remodeling. *PLoS ONE*, 2015, 10(2), e0117110. doi:10.1371/journal.pone.0117110.

[353] FDA. FDA warns that gadolinium-based contrast agents (GBCAs) are retained in the body; requires new class warnings; 2017.

In: Horizons in World Cardiovascular … ISBN: 978-1-53616-157-1
Editor: Eleanor H. Bennington

Chapter 2

INFERIOR VENA CAVA (IVC) FILTERS

Husameddin El Khudari MD, Khalid Mahmoud MD, Andrew Gunn, MD, Aliaksei Salei, MD and Ahmed Kamel Abdel Aal*, MD, PhD

Division of Interventional Radiology, Department of Radiology
University of Alabama at Birmingham, UAB
Birmingham, AL, US

BACKGROUND

Venous thromboembolism (VTE) is a spectrum of disease that includes both deep venous thrombosis (DVT) and pulmonary embolism (PE). VTE affects 950,000 patients every year, including 500,000 new cases of acute DVT. DVT and acute PE are associated with significant morbidity and mortality. For example, every year 60,000 to 100,000 Americans die from VTE/PE, and PE is the third most common cause of cardiovascular death. 10% of PE are fatal within 1 hour, and 5-10% of patients present in shock. Up to 60% of patients with acute DVT will develop post-thrombotic syndrome (PTS).

* Corresponding Author's Email: akamel@uabmc.edu.

Risk Factors for VTE

Risk factors can be classified into strong, moderate and weak factors. Strong risk factors have an odds ratio >10, and include major trauma, major surgery, spinal cord injury, hip or leg fracture, and hip or knee replacement. Moderate risk factors have an odds ratio of 2-9, and include malignancy, thrombophilia, previous thromboembolism, pregnancy, post-partum state, hormone replacement therapy, paralytic stroke, congestive heart failure and central venous lines. Low risk factors have an odd ratio <2, and include obesity, age >40, prolonged sitting (car or air travel), laparoscopic surgery and varicose veins.

Hereditary risk factors for VTE include factor V Leiden deficiency, protein C and Protein S deficiencies, activated protein C resistance, factor II (prothrombin) G20210A mutation, and Anti-thrombin deficiency.

Management of VTE

The mainstay of therapy for DVT is anticoagulation. The aim is to prevent PE, reduce PTS, improve short term and long term quality of life and reduce the risk of recurrent DVT. Inferior vena cava interruption represents an alternative when anticoagulation fails or is contraindicated.

IVC Interruption

Surgical interruption of the IVC for the prevention of PE was first performed in 1893. Surgical interruption took many forms such as ligation, plication, clipping, or stapling. IVC thrombosis was a frequent complication after these surgeries. Endovascular or trans-venous IVC interruption became clinically feasible in 1967 after the introduction of the Mobin-Uddin filter. Many percutaneous IVC filters have since been developed.

INFERIOR VENA CAVA FILTERS

Inferior vena cava (IVC) filters are interruption devices and their placement provide an alternative option to anticoagulation. Filters do not prevent the development of VTE. In fact, filters are strongly believed to increase the long-term risk of DVT without influencing overall mortality from VTE. The PREPIC Trial in 2005 is the only randomized study that compared anticoagulation alone to anticoagulation plus IVC filter. In the trial, 400 patients were followed for 8 years. The conclusion was that filters reduced the risk of PE but increased that of DVT and had no effect on survival. Although their use may be beneficial in patients at high risk of PE, systematic use in the general population with VTE is not recommended.

Indications

The major consensus indications for IVC filter placement are an existence of absolute contraindication to therapeutic anticoagulation, complication related to anticoagulation, and acute proximal venous thrombosis despite anticoagulation. In addition, it is often used as adjunctive therapy for recurrent PE in patients who are on anticoagulants or in patients with poor tolerance to additional embolic events due to their medical comorbidities.

In general indications can be divided into absolute, relative and prophylactic.

a. *Absolute indications:*
   - Venous Thromboembolism (VTE) with contraindication to anticoagulation
   - Failure of anticoagulation (Recurrent VTE despite adequate anticoagulation
   - Inability to achieve or to maintain anticoagulation
   - Complications of anticoagulation

b. *Relative indications*:
   - Large, free floating thrombus
   - Thromboembolic disease with limited cardiopulmonary reserve
   - Recurrent PE despite primary therapy
   - DVT thrombolysis. Massive PE treated with thrombolysis/ thrombectomy
   - Chronic Pulmonary Embolism (PE) treated with thrombo-endarterectomy
   - Iliocaval DVT
   - Thrombolysis for iliocaval DVT
   - Difficulty establishing therapeutic anticoagulation
   - Recurrent PE with filter in place
   - Poor compliance with anticoagulant medications
   - High risk of complication of anticoagulation (e.g., ataxia, frequent falls)

c. *Prophylactic indications:*

   The patient does not have VTE, however is at increased risk for development of clinically significant PE, or is unable to undergo primary prophylaxis. This includes;
   - Trauma or post-surgical patient with high risk of VTE
   - Surgical procedure in patient at high risk of VTE
   - Closed head injury
   - Spinal cord injury
   - Multiple long-bone or pelvic fractures
   - Medical condition with high risk of VTE (e.g., immobilized or in an intensive care unit)

However, there is discrepancy and variability in the indications for IVC filter placement based on societies' guidelines. Some of the variability appears to be related to scarcity of available evidence. This might also be augmented by the differences in the interpretation of these guidelines by the operating and requesting physicians. This is mostly noticed in patients who had contraindication to or failure of anticoagulation, and when prophylactic filter placement is requested. As an example of the later, the Eastern Association for the Surgery of Trauma (EAST) guidelines suggest prophylactic IVC filter use in high-risk patients, but the American College of Chest Physicians (ACCP) guidelines do not.

Contraindications

There are only a few contraindications for IVC filter placement. These include:

a. *Absolute contraindications:*
   - Occlusion or absence of the IVC, which preclude filter placement.
   - Lack of venous access to the IVC (occluded internal jugular, subclavian and femoral veins).

b. *Relative contraindications:*
   - Allergy to iodinated contrast media and renal insufficiency (CO2 or gadolinium can be used instead).
   - Uncorrectable severe coagulopathy.
   - Bacteremia or untreated infections

IDEAL IVC FILTER

The ideal IVC filter should have a number of characteristics, which include:

- Non-thrombogenic and biocompatible, with infinite implant life
- High filtering efficiency (large and small emboli) without impedance of flow
- Secure fixation to the IVC wall with no migration or tilting
- Ease of percutaneous insertion

- Small delivery system
- Potentially amenable to repositioning
- Magnetic resonance imaging compatibility.
- Low cost
- Low access site thrombosis
- Ease and efficacy of retrievability

TYPES OF IVC FILTERS

There are three common IVC filters designs; conical (umbrella), hexagon double basket and helical. There are two types of IVC filters; optional (retrievable and convertible), and permanent. The retrievable filters were introduced in the late 1990's, allowing the filter removal once the risk of VTE has resolved.

Retrievable IVC Filter

There are currently many available retrievable IVC filters which include:

- Denali (Bard Peripheral Vascular, Tempe, AZ)
- Celect (Cook Medical, Bloomington, IN)
- Günther Tulip (Cook Medical)
- Eclipse (Bard Peripheral Vascular, Tempe, AZ)
- G2 (Bard Peripheral Vascular)
- G2X (G2 modified with hook, Bard Peripheral Vascular)
- Option (Argon Medical Devices, Inc. Plano, TX)
- OptEase (Cordis Corporation, Bridgewater, NJ)
- Crux (Volcano Corporation, San Diego, CA)
- ALN filter (ALN Implants Chirurgicaux, Ghisonaccia, France)

Retrievable filters are made of stainless steel, nitinol, titanium, or conichrome. They have design elements that allow retrieval. These include flexible and smaller hooks, filter collapsibility and flexibility, and unrestrained anchor legs, as well as other elements. These design modifications have placed some optional filters at risk for fatigue and failure resulting in fracture, migration, and IVC wall penetration or perforation. Most of the optional filters can be placed in an IVC up to 30 mm in diameter, except for the ALN filter which can be placed up to 32 mm, and the Crux and Denali filters which can only be placed in up to 28 mm maximum IVC diameter. Currently, there are no definite guidelines on the time to retrieve these filters, and poor clinical follow-up plays an important role in low retrieval rates.

Convertible IVC Filters

A few convertible filters are available for clinical use. The VenaTech Convertible filter (B. Braun Interventional Systems, Inc, Bethlehem, Pennsylvania) is an example of these filters. The filter has a conical design that safely captures and assists in dissolving trapped thrombus in the filter cone. When further filtering is no longer needed, a conversion procedure can be performed using a snare by capturing the hook on the cone of the filter and pulling it proximally until the filter head unlocks. The filtering mechanism will be deactivated and the filter will be converted to open configuration. After conversion, endothelialization of the filter struts occurs over time, and the filter essentially becomes an IVC stent. In a recent multicenter trial on the VenaTech Convertible filter, the filter was placed successfully in 149 patients. One migration to the right atrium required surgical removal. Technical success rate for filter conversion was 92.7%. Mean time from placement to conversion was 130.7 days (range, 15–391 days). No major conversion-related events were reported. The mean conversion procedure time was 30.7 minutes (range, 7–135 min). There were 89 converted and 32 unconverted patients who completed 6-month follow-up with no delayed complications. This study shows that the VenaTech

Convertible filter has a high conversion rate and low 6-month device-related adverse events. Yet, further studies are necessary to determine long-term safety and efficacy in both converted and unconverted patients.

A second example of convertible filters is the Sentry bio-convertible IVC filter (BTG International Inc, London, United Kingdom). It is designed to provide temporary protection against PE during transient high-risk periods. Bioconversion refers to hydrolytic degradation of the bio-absorbable filament which lead to the release of filter arms from the filtering cone in the central portion of the IVC lumen, therefore avoiding the need for a second (retrieval or conversion) intervention and leaving a patent IVC lumen. In its one-year analysis, the prospective multicenter SENTRY clinical trial found that clinical success was achieved in 111 of 114 evaluable patients. The rate of freedom from new symptomatic PE at 60 days was 100%, and there were no cases of PE at 12 months for either therapeutic or prophylactic indications. Two patients (1.6%) developed symptomatic caval thrombosis during the first month; neither experienced recurrence after successful interventions. There was no filter tilting, migration, embolization, fracture, or caval perforation by the filter, and no filter-related death through 12 months. Filter bioconversion was successful with a rate of 95.7% (110/115) at 6 months and 96.4% (106/110) at 12 months.

Permanent IVC Filters

Several permanent filters are available including:

- Greenfield stainless-steel filter and titanium filter (Boston Scientific)
- VenaTech LGM and LP filters (B Braun)
- Gianturco–Roehm Bird's Nest filter (Cook)
- TrapEase filter (Cordis)
- Simon nitinol filter (Bard)

Most of the permanent filters can only be placed in an IVC with a diameter of 28 mm or less. TrapEase can be used up to 30 mm. Bird's Nest filter can be placed in an IVC with up to a diameter of 40 mm.

Both permanent and optional filters have similar efficacy and safety profiles. In fact, any optional filter may become permanent due to many factors, such as a change in the patient's clinical status, lack of follow-up, or inability to retrieve the filter. Thus, the existing indications for permanent filters are applicable to optional filters.

IVC Filter Placement Technique

Pre-Procedure Care

A careful review of the history, physical exam and laboratory findings is important to ensure a valid indication for IVC filter placement. The platelet count should be >50,000, and the INR should be less than 2. Evaluation of the creatinine level, white blood cell count and previously obtained cultures is recommended. Available cross-sectional imaging should be reviewed for vena caval anomalies, presence of an IVC thrombus, extrinsic compression, the level of renal veins inflow, any left renal vein variants, and the IVC size if possible. The access site should also be evaluated in the available imaging.

Technique of Placement

The procedure is usually performed under moderate sedation with monitoring of the patient's heart rate, cardiac rhythm, and blood pressure by a dedicated healthcare provider. Sonographic examination of the access site is preferably performed to assess the patency and caliber of the internal jugular or the femoral veins. A right-sided approach, regardless of access vessel, is generally preferred over the left side given the more direct route to the IVC. After obtaining venous access, a 5 Fr pigtail catheter or the filter placement kit sheath is then advanced into the left common iliac vein (with jugular access), or into the ipsilateral common iliac vein (with femoral access). An inferior vena cavogram is then performed to evaluate IVC caliber, presence of filling defects within the IVC, presence of variant anatomy and to locate the inflow of the renal veins (Figure 1).

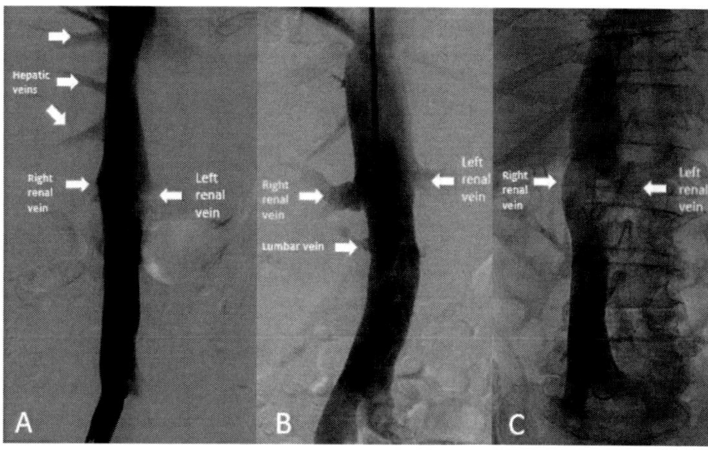

Figure 1. (a) Femoral, (b) and (c) Jugular access in three different patients. In (a) and (b) the filter placement sheath was used for the inferior vena cavogram. In (c) the pigtail catheter was used and placed in the left iliac vein.

If the diameter of the cava is too large on the anteroposterior (AP) projection, then a lateral cavogram can be obtained. The filter can be carefully placed if the diameter obtained from the lateral cavogram is appropriate. Absence of left common iliac vein inflow on the cavogram may be seen in caval duplication, left pelvic DVT, and May-Thurner syndrome. The filter is then advanced through the sheath and positioned in the infra-renal IVC (unless there is an indication for a suprarenal filter placement). The filter is then deployed with the apex of the filter at or slightly above the lower edge of the orifice of the lowest renal vein (Figure 2). This positioning will allow the renal inflow to clear clot from the filter apex. If a thrombus is detected on the inferior vena cavogram, the filter should be placed above the most cranial extension of the thrombus. If the thrombus extends to the level of the renal vein, then the filter should be placed in the suprarenal IVC. Positioning can be confirmed fluoroscopically and by a repeat inferior vena cavogram.

Care should be practiced to recognize inadvertent cannulation of the right gonadal vein that can occur with jugular access. The right gonadal vein usually enters the IVC just inferior to the right renal vein and has a course that is parallel and just lateral to the IVC (Figure 3).

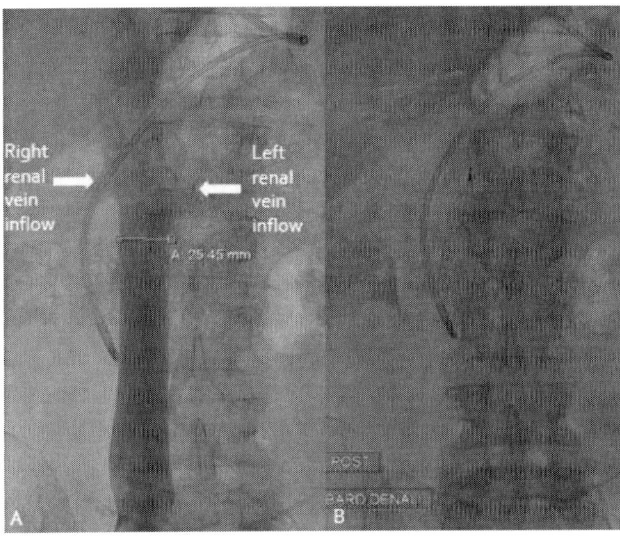

Figure 2. (a) Inferior vena cavogram showing renal veins inflow and an IVC diameter of 25 mm. (b) Bard Denali filter placed in appropriate position with the apex slightly above the renal veins' inflow.

Alternatively, IVC filters can be placed at the bedside either using fluoroscopy or transabdominal or intravascular ultrasound. This is usually done for ICU patients whose condition is critical that transportation to the angiosuite poses a risk.

Suprarenal Filter Placement

Suprarenal caval filter placement may be considered when any of the following situations exist:

- Presence of IVC thrombus precluding placement of a filter in the infrarenal IVC (Figure 4);

- Filter placement during pregnancy (suprarenal placement is also appropriate in women of childbearing age);
- Thrombus extending above previously placed infrarenal filter;
- Gonadal vein thrombosis;
- Anatomic variants, e.g., duplication of the IVC, low insertion of renal veins;
- Significant extrinsic compression of the infrarenal IVC;
- Intrinsic narrowing of the infrarenal IVC;
- Intraabdominal or pelvic mass in patients who will undergo surgery and in whom operative IVC mobilization is contemplated.

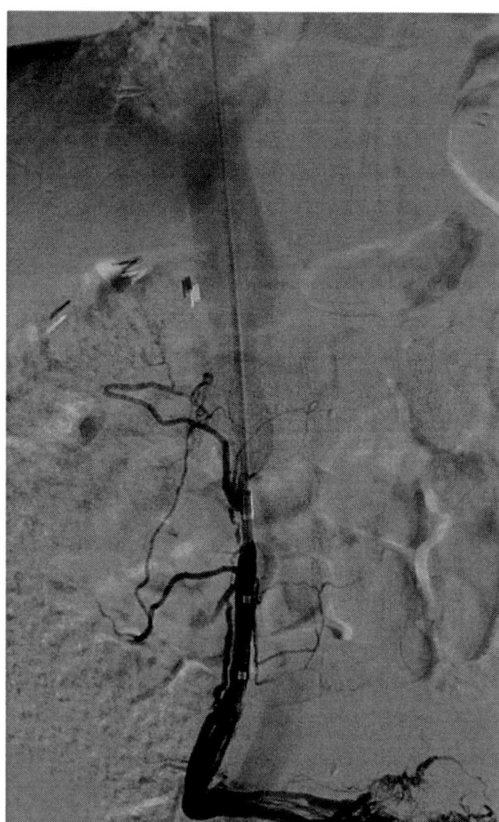

Figure 3. Inadvertent catheterization of the right gonadal vein during IVC filter placement.

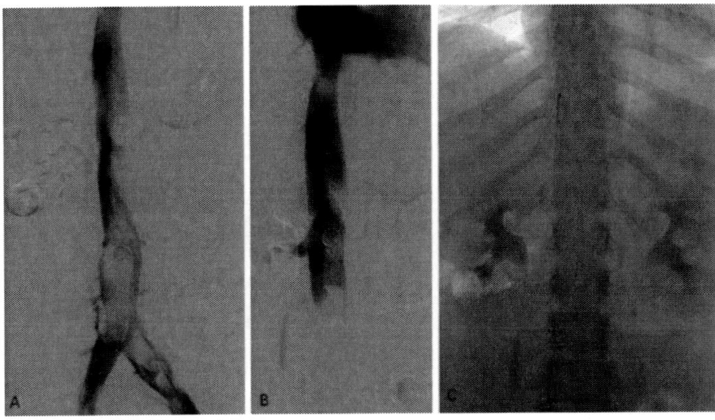

Figure 4. (a) Inferior vena cavogram showing thrombus in the infrarenal IVC. (b) Inferior vena cavogram showing patent suprarenal IVC. (c) Placement of filter in the suprarenal IVC.

Duplicated IVC

The prevalence of this variant is 1%. The two IVCs usually join at the left renal vein (Figure 5a). In these cases, one IVC filter can be placed in each IVC below each renal vein (Figure 5b). Alternatively, a single suprarenal filter can be placed. If the duplicated IVC is accessory with a small caliber, it can be embolized and a filter is placed in the main IVC.

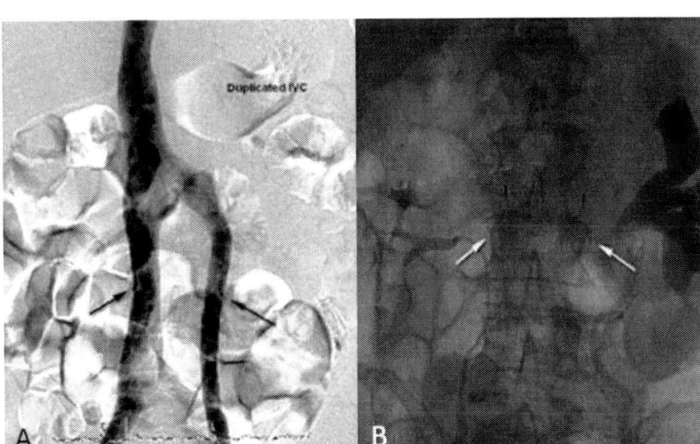

Figure 5. (a) Inferior vena cavogram showing duplicated IVC. (b) 2 IVC filters placed, one in each IVC.

Circumaortic Left Renal Vein

The prevalence of this variant is 3-8%. The lower component runs behind the aorta and drains into the IVC at a lower level than the normal left renal vein (Figure 6a). The main concern here is if the filter is placed between the two veins, embolization can occur around the venous ring (Figure 6b). The IVC filter should be placed below the orifice of the retrocaval component, or in a suprarenal location.

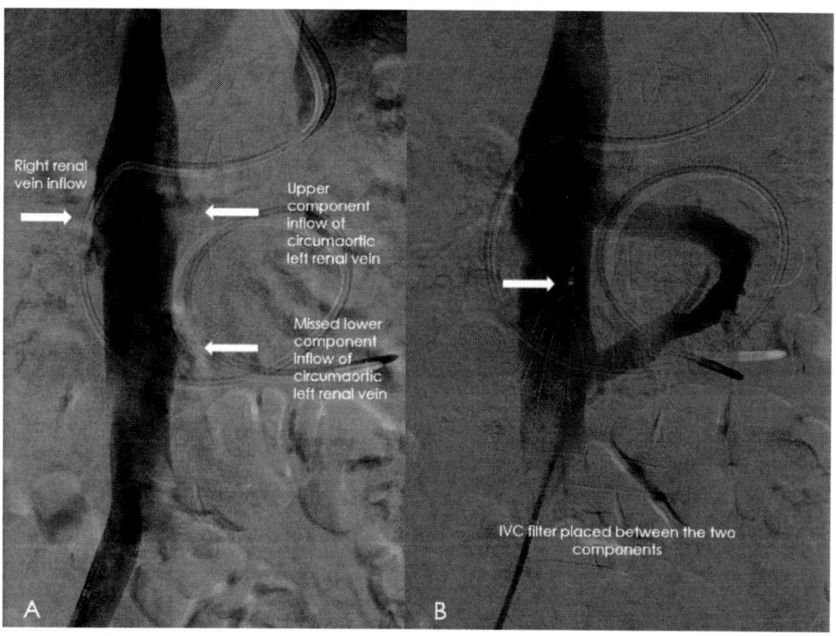

Figure 6. (a) Inferior vena cavogram showing right renal vein inflow and circumaortic left renal vein inflow that was misinterpreted as a single left renal inflow at L1 level. (b) Inferior vena cavogram after filter placement clearly showed the circumaortic left renal vein with the filter positioned above the lower component, with risk of embolization through the venous ring. The misplaced filter was removed.

Retroaortic Left Renal Vein

The prevalence of this variant is 2-3%. The left renal vein drains into the IVC below the right renal vein or sometimes at the confluence of the iliac veins. The IVC filter should be placed below the orifice of the left renal vein if there is enough space in the IVC (Figures 7 and 8), otherwise the filter can be placed with the apex at the level of the right renal vein or one filter can be placed in each common iliac vein.

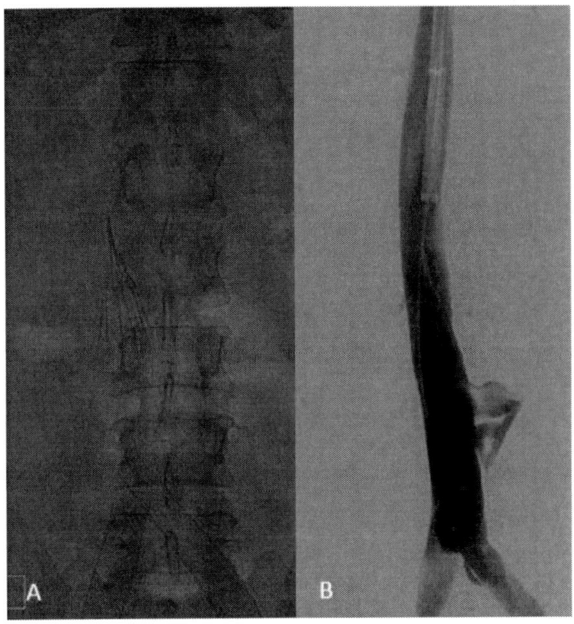

Figure 7. (a) IVC filter placed at an outside hospital. (b) Inferior vena cavogram showing a left retroaortic renal vein below the level of the filter.

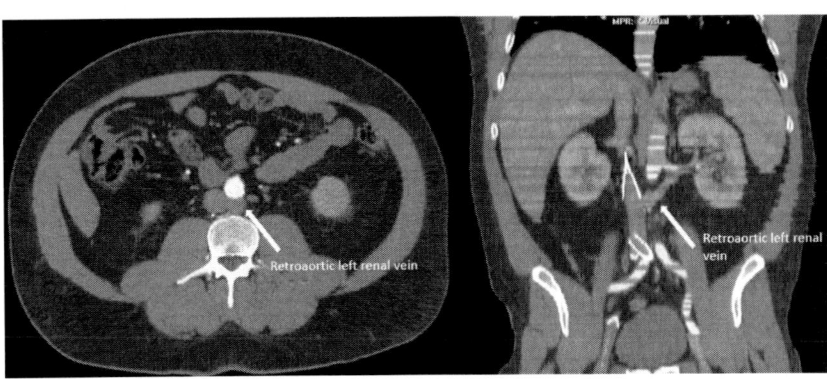

Figure 8. CT scan of the abdomen at outside hospital. (a) Axial and (b) coronal images showing retroaortic left renal vein.

Megacava

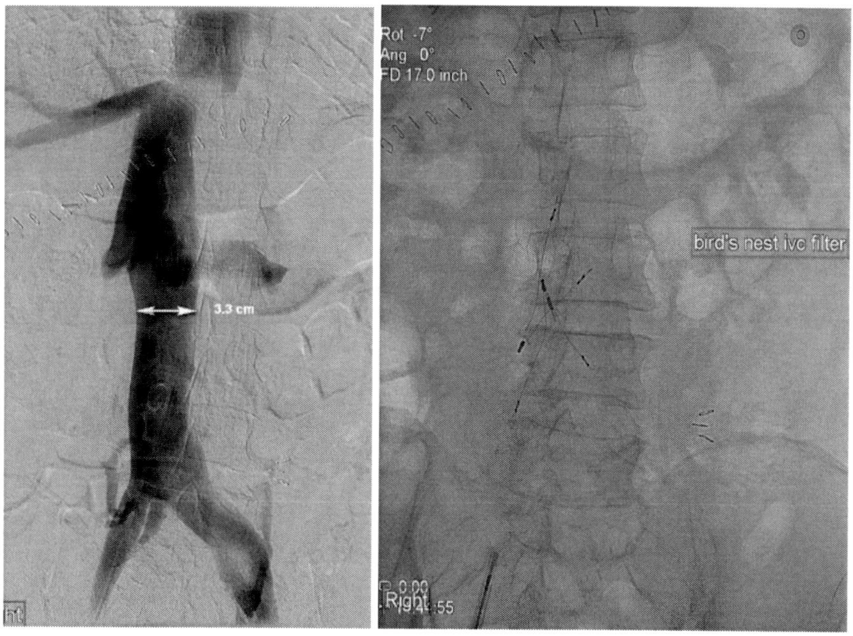

Figure 9. (a) Inferior vena cavogram showing megacava measuring up to 3.3 cm, (b) Bird's nest IVC filter placed.

If the IVC diameter is greater than 28 mm, it is called a megacava (Figure 9a). The incidence of megacava is <1%. Gianturco–Roehm Bird's Nest filter (Cook) can be used in vena cava measuring up to 40 mm in diameter (Figure 9b). Alternatively, one IVC filter can be placed in each common iliac vein.

Left Sided IVC

The prevalence of this variant is 0.2%–0.5%. Similar to a duplicated IVC, a left-sided IVC courses cranially to the left of the abdominal aorta, joins with the left renal vein, and drains into a normal suprarenal IVC.

Post-Procedure Care

Following IVC filter placement, the patient should be on bed rest and observed in the initial post-procedure period; the length of bed rest depends on the approach, the size of the venotomy and the patient's medical condition. For patients with jugular filter placement, the head of the bed should be elevated to 45 degrees or more for approximately four hours. If the patient has had the filter placed from a femoral approach, most patients will remain on bed rest for four hours with the access leg straight. Initial ambulation of the patient must be supervised. Documentation of complete recovery from sedation is required. The patient should be made aware of potential issues related future venous cannulation that may dislodge the filter or lead to guidewire entrapment.

Whether to anticoagulate the patient following IVC filter placement if the contraindication to anticoagulation has resolved is controversial. Some patient populations are at increased risk for thrombosis (e.g., patients with malignancy) such that initiating anticoagulation, if feasible, may reduce the rate of filter-related thrombosis. This decision should be made on an individualized patient by patient basis.

IVC Filter Complications

Indwelling IVC filters can result in complications including filter penetration of adjacent viscera (e.g., duodenum, liver, pancreas, ureter) (Figure 10), adjacent vessel perforation (e.g., aorta, lumbar artery, renal artery, common iliac artery) (Figure 11), displacement or migration, tilt, device fracture and thrombosis. The risk of complications increases with longer dwell times.

A review of the U.S. Food and Drug Administration's (FDA's) Manufacturer and User Facility Device Experience (MAUDE) database found that 87% of user-reported events were attributable to optional IVC filters, whereas 13% were associated with permanent devices.

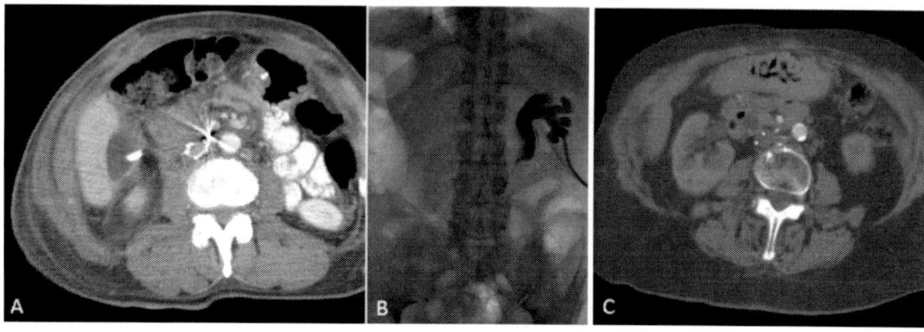

Figure 10. (a) Axial CT scan image showing penetration of one of the IVC filter struts into the right ureter causing hydronephrosis. (b) Nephrostogram showing obstruction of the proximal right ureter by penetrating IVC filter strut causing ureteral stricture. (C) Axial CT scan image showing penetration of one of the filter struts into the vertebral body.

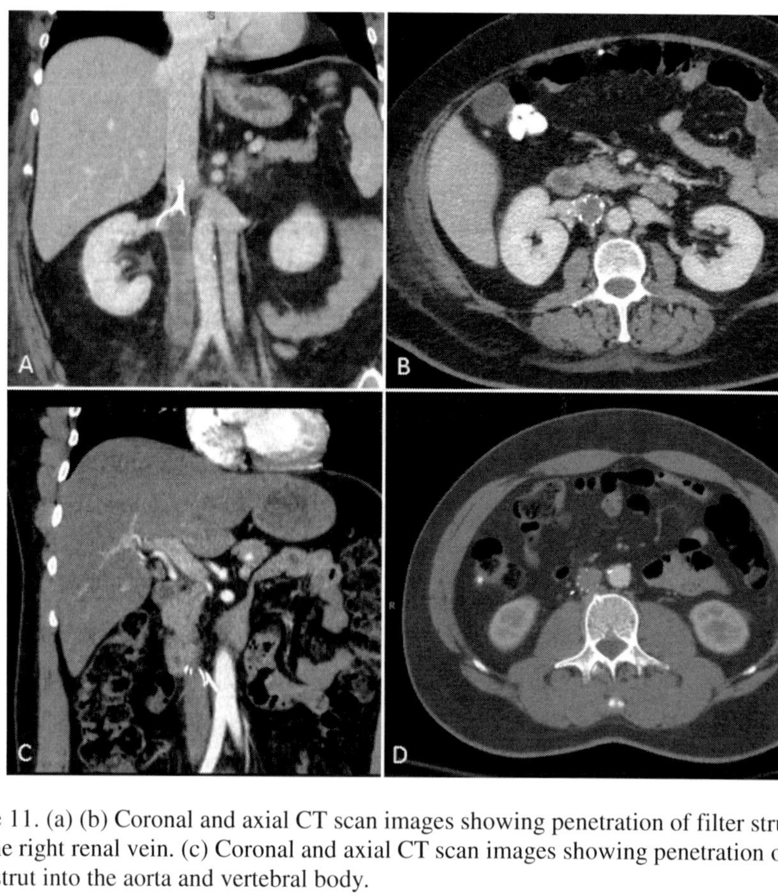

Figure 11. (a) (b) Coronal and axial CT scan images showing penetration of filter strut into the right renal vein. (c) Coronal and axial CT scan images showing penetration of filter strut into the aorta and vertebral body.

IVC filter complications can be divided into procedural complications, delayed complications and complications related to filter retrieval. Procedural complications are by far the most common.

Procedural Complications

- Venous Access Site: Occurs in up to 25% of the cases and includes bleeding, hematoma, inadvertent arterial puncture, infection, venous thrombosis and arteriovenous fistula.
- Malposition of the deployed filter: Occurs in 1-9% of cases.
- Defective Filter Deployment: Occurs in up to 23% of cases and include incomplete filter opening, non-target deployment, incomplete IVC expansion, crossed legs, and acute strut perforation.
- Pericardial tamponade for superior vena cava placement: Occurs in 2% of cases.
- IVC perforation (defined as a strut or anchor device extending >3mm outside the caval wall by CT, venography, or autopsy): Acute penetration occurring during placement of the filter is considered an insertion complication.
- Allergic reaction to contrast media or other medications.
- Entrapment of the guidewire within the filter.

Delayed Complications

- Migration: this is defined as movement >2cm away from the location of initial deployment. Filter or filter fragments migrating into the right atrium, pulmonary artery, right gonadal vein, lumbar veins, and even into the aorta have been reported. Major filter migration occurs in <1% of cases.
- Iliocaval thrombosis

- Filter Fracture: this is defined as any loss of a filter's structural integrity (i.e., breakage or separation) documented by imaging or at autopsy. It occurs in < 1% of cases.
- IVC Perforation: This is defined as a strut or anchor device extending >3mm outside the caval wall by CT, venography, or autopsy. It occurs in <1% of cases. Perforation of the caval wall by filter components is frequently encountered at cross-sectional imaging; however, the overall significance and magnitude of this issue remain an active area of debate.
- Pulmonary embolism
- Filter embolization: This is defined as post deployment movement of the filter or its components to a distant anatomic site.
- Device infection

FILTER RETRIEVAL

The rate of filter placement has increased rapidly until 2010. In 2010, the FDA recommended that "implanting physicians and clinicians responsible for the ongoing care of patients with retrievable IVC filters should consider removing the filter as soon as protection from PE is no longer needed". IVC filter placement has significantly declined nationally since the FDA advisory was released. Although the overall numbers have declined, the proportion of IVC filter placements in patients with VTE is increasing, suggesting a pivot towards more conservative absolute indications.

Patients with optional vena cava filters require routine follow-up and tracking to assess for filter retrieval. The decision of when to remove the filter varies for each device and patient condition. An acceptably low risk of clinically significant PE (which should be less than the risk of leaving the filter in place) is the most important criterion to consider filter retrieval. This could be achieved by starting and maintaining the patient on anticoagulation or by changes in the clinical condition of the patient which lowers the risk of developing VTE. After counseling, patients who desire to continue caval filtration permanently may do so. During the last decade, many centers aimed to improve their protocols to retrieve IVC filters for indicated candidates. For example, the rate of filter retrieval in our center improved significantly from 6.6% to 28.3%, ($p=0.00024$) within 9 months after introducing a policy of dedicated follow-up.

Indications for Filter Retrieval

An absolute indication for filter retrieval is a documented filter complication leading to major morbidity, e.g., a strut perforation causing severe pain.

Relative indications for filter removal are the resolution of the reason for filter placement. However, before deciding whether or not to retrieve an IVC filter, the following questions should be answered; what is the filter type? when was the filter placed? what was the indication? is the patient on anticoagulation? is the patient compliant with medications and follow ups? are there any signs of new, progressive or recurrent VTE? and are there any indications for permanent filtration in this patient?

The following criteria/conditions should be met:

A. The patient is at acceptably low risk of clinically significant PE.
B. The patient is compliant with medications and follow up.
C. The patient's life expectancy should be greater than 6 months, so that the potential benefits of discontinuation of filtration can be achieved.
D. The return to high risk VTE status is unlikely (e.g., interruption of anticoagulant treatment for surgery, change in clinical management, or change in clinical condition).
E. The patient desires filter removal or conversion.

Patients with documented VTE should be on therapeutic anticoagulation for at least 2-3 weeks (symptomatic PE is most likely to occur within 2 to 3 weeks after initiation of anticoagulation), and should have no clinical evidence of progressive VTE (no evidence of anticoagulation failure or complications of anticoagulation). In provoked VTE, if the patient is no longer at risk for VTE, the filter should be removed. Patients without documented VTE (prophylactic indications), should be either on prophylactic anticoagulation or the risk factors for DVT has resolved before filter removal is considered. A patient who develops VTE while a prophylactic filter is in place should be managed with primary therapy for VTE. Prior to filter retrieval, a complete blood count and coagulation profile may be needed for patients on anticoagulation. Renal function tests should be considered for patients at risk for contrast induced nephropathy.

Patients should be managed according to their VTE status after retrieval or conversion of a filter. Patients with a diagnosis of VTE should be treated for the full duration suggested in published practice guidelines or according to local standards of care. Patients without VTE but who are still at risk may need prophylactic anticoagulation. After discontinuation of filtration, patients should be monitored for new, recurrent, or progressive DVT and/or PE, and, if diagnosed, managed accordingly.

Retrieval Techniques

Filter retrieval can be classified into standard techniques and advanced (complex) techniques. Generally, filter retrieval is done under moderate sedation, with general anesthesia reserved for complex cases.

Standard Technique

In general, conical filters have a hook at the apex directed upwards, including the Günther Tulip and Celect filters (Cook Medical, Bloomington, IN); the Recovery G2, G2X, and Eclipse filters (Bard Peripheral Vascular, Tempe, AZ), the Option filter (AngioTech, Vancouver, BC); and ALN filter (ALN Implants Chirurgicaux, Ghisonaccia, France). These are generally removed with an endovascular snare via jugular venous access (Figure 12).

The exception to this is the OptEase filter (Cordis Corporation, Bridgewater, NJ) which has a femoral retrieval kit, since the hook faces downwards (Figure 13). When these classical techniques fail, then advanced/complex techniques become necessary.

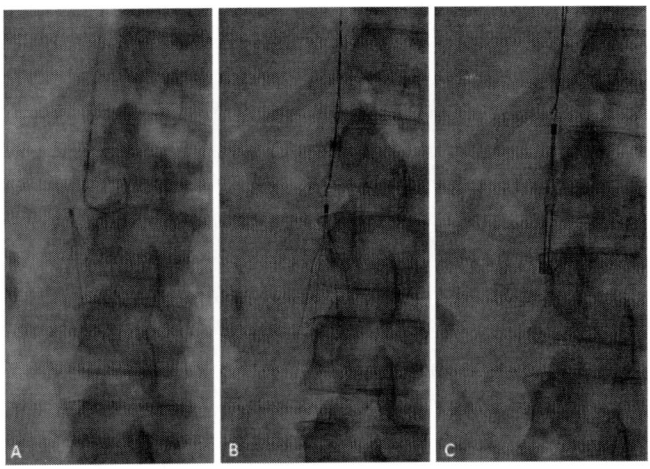

Figure 12. Standard retrieval technique. (a) Loop snare superior to the filter hook. (b) Engagement of the filter hook by the loop snare. (c) Advancement of the sheath over the filter followed by retracting the filter out.

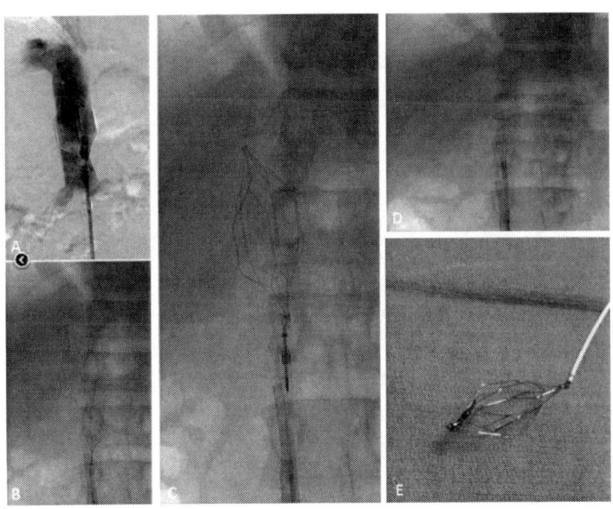

Figure 13. Standard technique for retrieval of OptEase filter. (a) Inferior vena cavogram showing suprarenal filter with no clots. (b) En-Snare close to the hook at the inferior aspect of the filter. (c) Engagement of the filter hook by the snare. (d) Retraction of the filter into the sheath. (e) Photo of the retrieved filter engaged by the snare.

Advanced Techniques

Most of the difficulties encountered during standard removal techniques can be overcome with the use of certain advanced retrieval techniques. However, it is important to realize that aggressive attempts at filter retrieval may be associated with increased risks of complications, including access site complications secondary to the use of large sheath size, intra-procedural caval thrombosis or vasospasm, and the potential for caval injury and hemorrhage. These concerns should be carefully weighed against the long-term risks of indwelling filters.

Both filter tilt and female gender are associated with the need for advanced retrieval techniques.

Advanced techniques include:

Single Access Techniques

1. Realignment Technique

Angled Catheter-Snare Technique

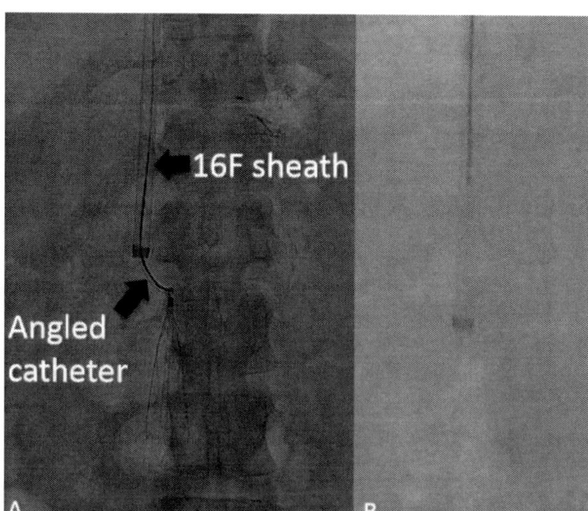

Figure 14: (a) Angled catheter is used to snare the filter hook and align it with the sheath. (b) The filter was retrieved through the sheath.

This technique uses the endovascular loop snare to grasp the tilted IVC filter. An angled catheter is used to redirect the snare toward the filter tip which then allows central orientation of the filter into the vascular sheath. (Figure 14).

2. Displacement Techniques

Stiff Wire Displacement Technique

This technique uses a stiff wire to straighten the tilted IVC filter. The wire is advanced between the caval wall and filter apex to displace the IVC filter away from the caval wall. This allows the endovascular snare to capture the filter hook. Then, the filter can be removed.

Balloon Displacement Technique

This technique can be used with single access or with dual access. Again, a wire is advanced in between the caval wall and the filter apex. Once in position, an interposed angioplasty balloon can be used to displace the tilted filter by inflating it between the filter struts and apex. This allows the endovascular snare to capture the filter hook. Then, the filter can be removed

Curved Catheter Twist Technique

This technique can be used to center a tilted filter. A curved catheter is directed around the superior aspect of the filter cone. By twisting the catheter, an attempt to center the tilted filter is made. An additional tug on the catheter may force the filter to center. When the filter hook has been centered or adequately shifted away from the wall, the filter can then be retrieved in conventional fashion. In this technique, it is important to avoid engaging the secondary struts. Additionally, excessive twisting of the catheter should be avoided, as this could cause damage to the catheter and may prevent its safe removal. If there is a lack of filter movement despite twisting and gentle tugging, this technique should be abandoned.

3. Sling Techniques

Wire Loopsnare Technique

In case of an embedded IVC filter apex, this technique is used. A reverse-curve catheter is guided through the filter struts and a hydrophilic wire is advanced through the catheter cranially. Then, the endovascular snare grasps the wire to create a wire loopsnare underneath the filter apex. The filter can then be removed through the sheath (Figure 15).

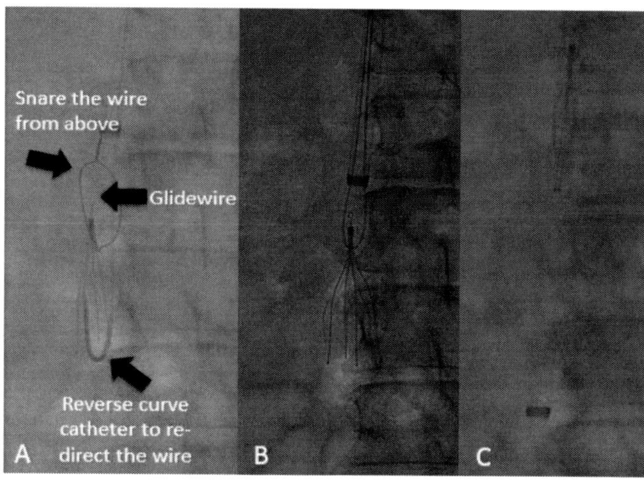

Figure 15. (a) Reversed curve catheter is used to direct a glide wire cranially through the filter apex. The glide wire is then snared and pulled into the jugular sheath. (b) The jugular sheath is the advanced to create an in-situ snare and align the filter to the sheath. (c) The filter is then retrieved.

Fibrin Cap Disruption Techniques

Due to turbulent blood flow, a fibrin cap can be formed at the filter apex and fix the apex to the caval wall. A modified technique that targets the fibrin cap can also be used. In this technique, a reverse-curve catheter is used to engage the radiolucent hyperplastic cap encasing the filter apex. This can be achieved by using the catheter to probe the IVC wall gently near the retrieval hook. Using fluoroscopic guidance and manual catheter feedback, the fibrin cap can be hooked with the catheter. A hydrophilic wire is then passed cranially and snared, forming a wire loop through the tissue cap. The sheath is then advanced coaxially, resulting in either capture and collapse of the filter or disruption of the tissue cap with subsequent use of standard retrieval techniques. The remnant of the tissue cap is frequently seen on the retrieved filter.

Dual-Access Techniques

These techniques are used when the single access techniques fail. Femoral and jugular access should be established to perform these techniques.

1. Wire and Snare Technique

The wire introduced through jugular access and directed between the caval wall and the filter apex, then the wire grasped by an endovascular snare from femoral access. Wire traction from both accesses performed simultaneously to displace the filter apex from the caval wall and align the filter with the retrieval sheath (Figure 16).

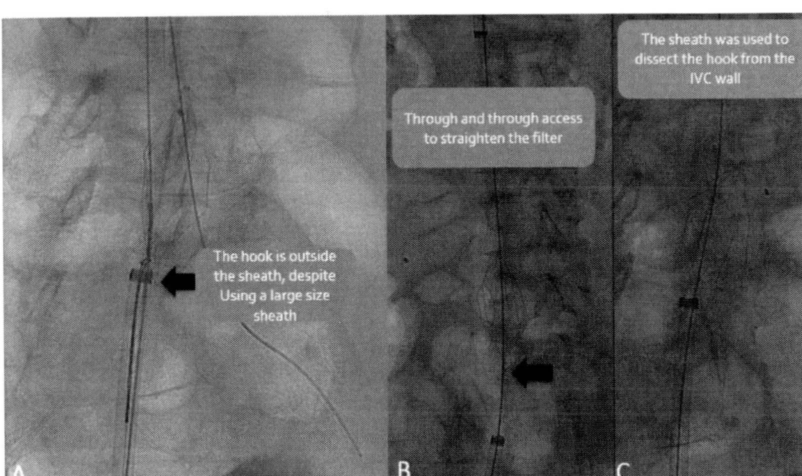

Figure 16. Wire and snare dual access technique.

2. Sandwich Technique

In this technique, two wires and two sheaths are used. The jugular access wire is directed between the caval wall and the filter apex and snared from below through the femoral access. The femoral access wire directed to the opposite side of the filter and snared from above through the jugular access. Then, both sheaths approached to the filter to apply traction on the filter from both ends, allowing it to collapse within one of the sheaths.

Dissection Techniques

These approaches dissect the filter away from the caval wall. Generally, they are more invasive than the aforementioned techniques due to the possible risk of IVC perforation.

1. Rigid Endobronchial Forceps

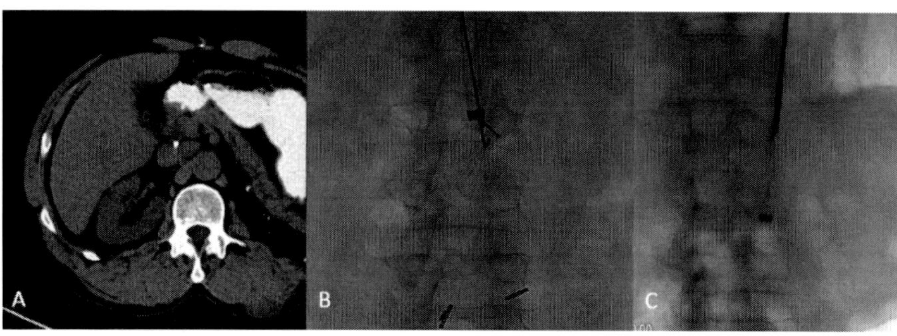

Figure 17. (a). Axial CT scan image showing embedded filter apex. (b)The filter apex is grasped using the endobronchial forceps. (c) The filter was sheathed and removed.

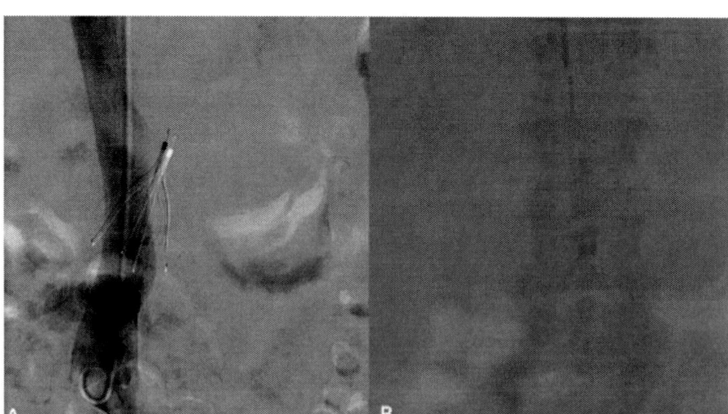

Figure 18: (a) inferior vena cavogram showing that the filter hook penetrated outside the caval wall. (b) The filter was retrieved using endobronchial forceps.

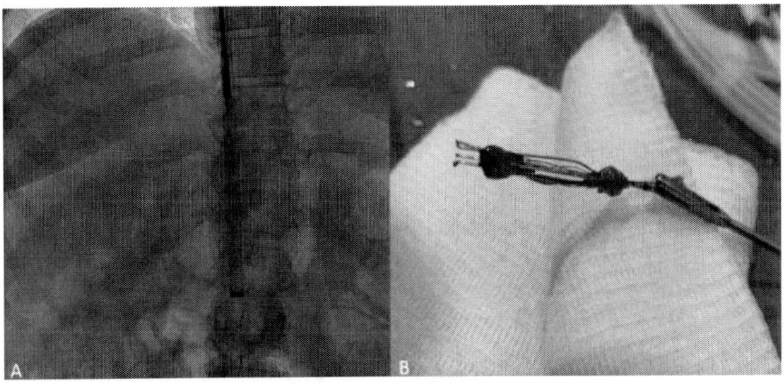

Figure 19. (a) Filter was retrieved using endobronchial forceps. (b) Photo of the retrieved filter.

This technique can be used to dissect tissue away from the filter apex. This allows either grasping the filter hook with an endovascular snare or retrieving the filter with the forceps themselves. This technique requires at least a 14 French vascular sheath (Figure 17, 18 and 19). Endobronchial forceps are malleable and can be shaped to provide the appropriate curvature to reach a tilted or embedded filter apex.

2. Laser Ablation

Laser ablation sheaths were originally designed for pacemaker lead extraction; however, they have been successfully used off-label to photothermally ablate neointimal tissue encasing the filter struts, allowing filter retrieval without the need to exert large, potentially hazardous forces. After grasping the filter hook with one of the aforementioned approaches, the laser sheath is sequentially activated to ablate the encasing tissue around the filter. The filter is then removed through the sheath.

Piecemeal Filter Extraction

This technique could be used as a last resort if all the other advanced techniques have failed. It includes the piecemeal extraction of the filter by means of intentional mechanical fracture of its components (Figure 20). This method carries a higher risk of filter component displacement and embolization.

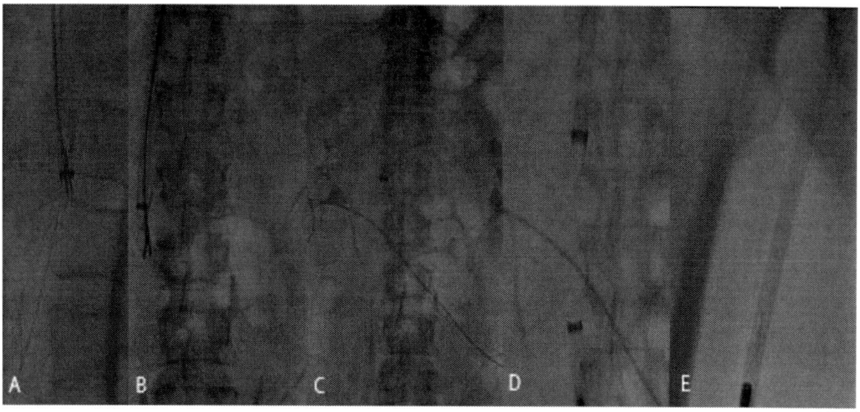

Figure 20. A through E show filter retrieval in pieces using both internal jugular and femoral access.

IVC Filter Retrieval Complications

Retrieval complications can include:

- Inability to retrieve the filter
- Intraprocedural caval thrombosis
- Hemorrhage
- Caval injury
- Filter fragment embolization
- IVC pseudoaneurysm

Reasons for Technical Failure during retrieval:

- Inability to grasp the hook of the filter due to filter tilt or embedment
- Dense adherence of the filter struts to the caval wall
- Longer dwell times
- History of caval thrombosis.

References

[1] Beckman, M., Hooper, W.C., Critchley, S., Ortel, T. (2010). Venous thromboembolism: a public health concern. *American Journal of Preventive Medicine* 2010, April, 38(4 Suppl): S495-501.

[2] Mobin-Uddin, K., Smith, P.E., Martinez, L.O., et al. (1967). A vena caval filter for the prevention of pulmonary embolus. *Surg Forum* 1967; 18:209–211.

[3] AndersonJr, F., Spencer, F. (2003). Factors for Venous Thromboembolism. *Circulation* June Vol. 107, No.23. June, 2003.

[4] Smouse, B. and Johar, A. (2010). Is Market Growth of Vena Cava Filters Justified? A review of indications, use, and market analysis. *Endovascular Today,* 2010-02, Pages 74-77.

[5] White, R., Geraghty, E.M., Brunson, A., et al. (2013). High variation between hospitals in vena cava filter use for venous thromboembolism. *JAMA Intern Med* 2013; 173:506.

[6] Kaufman, J. (2006). Guidelines for the Use of Optional (Retrievable and Convertible) Vena Cava Filters. A summary of the SIR multidisciplinary consensus statement. *Endovascular today*, september 2006.

[7] McClendon, J., O'Shaughnessy, B., Smith, T., et al. (2012). Comprehensive Assessment of Prophylactic Preoperative Inferior Vena Cava Filters for Major Spinal Reconstruction in Adults. *Spine.* 2012/06/01, 37(13):1122–1129.

[8] Kinney, T. (2006). Inferior Vena Cava Filters. *Seminars in Interventional Radiology,* 2006-09; 23(3): 230–239. doi: 10.1055/s-2006-948760

[9] PREPIC Study Group. Eight-year follow-up of patients with permanent vena cava filters in the prevention of pulmonary embolism: the PREPIC (Prevention du Risque d'Embolie Pulmonaire par Interruption Cave) randomized study. *Circulation* 2005;112(3):416–422.

[10] Minocha, J., Idakoji, I., Riaz, A., et al. (2010). Improving inferior vena cava filter retrieval rates: impact of a dedicated inferior vena cava filter clinic. *J Vasc Interv Radiol* 2010;21(12):1847–1851

[11] Marquess, J., Burke, C., Beecham, A., et al. (2008). Factors associated with failed retrieval of the Günther Tulip inferior vena cava filter. *J Vasc Interv Radiol* 2008;19(9):1321–1327.

[12] Geisbüsch, P., Benenati, J.F., Peña, C.S., et al. (2012). Retrievable inferior vena cava filters: factors that affect retrieval success. *Cardiovasc Intervent Radiol* 2012;35(5):1059–1065.

[13] McLoney, E., Krishnasamy, V., Castle, J., et al. (2013). Complications of Celect, Günther tulip, and Greenfield inferior vena cava filters on CT follow-up: a single-institution experience. *J Vasc Interv Radiol* 2013;24(11):1723–1729.

[14] Caplin, D., Nikolic, B., Kalva, S., et al. for the Society of Interventional Radiology Standards of Practice Committee. (2011). Quality Improvement Guidelines for the Performance of Inferior Vena Cava Filter Placement for the Prevention of Pulmonary Embolism. *J Vasc Interv Radiol* 2011; 22:1499–1506.

[15] Wadhwa, V., Trivedi, P.S., Chatterjee, K., et al. (2017). Decreasing IVC filter placements in the post-FDA warning era: Insights from 2005-2013 Nationwide Inpatient Database. *J Vasc Interv Radiol* 2017.

[16] DeRubertis, B. (2012). Advanced IVC Filter Retrieval Techniques Options when risks of permanent device implantation outweigh the potential complications of retrieval. *Endovascular Today,* November 2012.

[17] Dowell, J., Wagner, D., Elliott, E., et al. (2016). Factors Associated with Advanced Inferior Vena Cava Filter Removals: A Single-Center Retrospective Study of 203 Patients Over 7 Years. *CardioVascular and Interventional Radiology,* 2016, Volume 39, Number 2, Page 218.

[18] Iliescu, B., Haskal, Z. (2012). Advanced Techniques for Removal of Retrievable Inferior Vena Cava Filters. *CardioVascular and Interventional Radiology,* 2012, Volume 35, Number 4, Page 741.

[19] Rubenstein, L., Chun, A.K., Chew, M., Binkert, C.A. (2007). Loop-snare technique for difficult inferior vena cava filter retrievals. *J Vasc Interv Radiol* 2007;18(10):1315–1318.

[20] Esparaz, A., Ryu, R., Gupta, R., et al. (2012). Fibrin cap disruption: an adjunctive technique for inferior vena cava filter retrieval. *J Vasc Interv Radiol* 2012;23(9): 1233–1235.

[21] Desai, K., Lewandowski, R., Salem, R., et al. (2015). Retrieval of inferior vena cava filters with prolonged dwell time: a single center experience in 648 retrieval procedures. *JAMA Intern Med* 2015;175(9): 1572–1574.

[22] Kuo, W., Cupp, J. (2010). The excimer laser sheath technique for embedded inferior vena cava filter removal. *J Vasc Interv Radiol* 2010;21(12):1896–1899.

[23] Kuo, W., Odegaard, J., Rosenberg, J., Hofmann, L. (2013). Excimer laser-assisted removal of embedded inferior vena cava filters: a single-center prospective study. *Circ Cardiovasc Interv* 2013;6(5): 560–566.

[24] Gunn, A., Ertel, N. (2018). Endovascular Retrieval of a Migrated TrapEase Inferior Vena Cava Filter From the Right Atrium: A Brief Report and Literature Review. *Vascular and Endovascular Surgery,* February 20, 2018.

[25] Andreoli, J., Lewandowski, R., Vogelzang, R., Ryu, R. (2014). Comparison of complication rates associated with permanent and retrievable inferior vena cava filters: a review of the MAUDE database. *J Vasc Interv Radiol* 2014;25(8):1181–1185.

[26] Sella, D., Olderburg, W.A. (2014). Complications of inferior vena cava filters. *Semin Vasc Surg.* 2013;26(1):23-28.

[27] Bos, A., Tullius, T., Patel, M., et al. (2016). Indwelling and Retrieval Complications of Denali and Celect Infrarenal Vena Cava Filters. *J Vasc Interv Radiol,* 2016-07-01, Volume 27, Issue 7, Pages 1021-102.

[28] Bos, A., Van Ha, T., Van Beek, D., et al. (2015). Strut penetration: local complications, breakthrough pulmonary embolism, and retrieval failure in patients with Celect vena cava filters. *J Vasc Interv Radiol* 2015;26(1):101–106.

[29] Durack, J., Westphalen, A., Kekulawela, S., et al. (2012). Perforation of the IVC: rule rather than exception after longer indwelling times for the Günther Tulip and Celect retrievable filters. *Cardiovasc Intervent Radiol* 2012;35(2):299–308.

[30] Jia, Z., Wu, A., Tam, M., et al. (2015). Caval penetration by inferior vena cava filters: a systematic literature review of clinical significance and management. *Circulation* 2015;132 (10): 944–952.

[31] White, R., Geraghty, E.M., Brunson, A., et al. (2013). High variation between hospitals in vena cava filter use for venous thromboembolism. *JAMA Intern Med* 2013; 173:506.

[32] Ahmed, O., Hadied, M., Madassery, S. (2018). Retrieval of a permanent VenaTech LGM filter 18 years after implantation using a novel removal method. *Journal of Vascular Surgery: Venous and Lymphatic Disorder*s Volume 6, Issue 4, July 2018, Pages 526-529.

[33] Hohenwalter, E., Stone, J., O'Moore, P., et al. (2017). Multicenter Trial of the VenaTech Convertible Vena Cava Filter. *J Vasc Interv Radiol,* 2017-10-01, Volume 28, Issue 10, Pages 1353-1362.

[34] Dake, M., Murphy, T., Kramer, A., et al. One-Year Analysis of the Prospective Multicenter SENTRY Clinical Trial: Safety and Effectiveness of the Novate Sentry Bioconvertible Inferior Vena Cava Filter. *J Vasc Interv Radiol October* 2018 Volume 29, Issue 10, Pages 1350–1361.

[35] *http://www.bisusa.org/products/vena-cava-filters/vena-tech-lp-vena-cava-filter*

In: Horizons in World Cardiovascular … ISBN: 978-1-53616-157-1
Editor: Eleanor H. Bennington

Chapter 3

SUPERIOR MESENTERIC ARTERY SYNDROME: CLINICAL FEATURES, INVESTIGATIONS AND TREATMENTS

Adam G. Hague and Clive J. Kelty
Department of Upper Gastrointestinal Surgery,
Northern General Hospital, Herries Road, Sheffield, UK

ABSTRACT

Superior mesenteric artery (SMA) syndrome is a rare clinical entity. It results in partial or complete duodenal obstruction, due to compression of the third part of the duodenum between the superior mesenteric artery and the aorta. This is due to loss of the mesenteric fat pad. It can present acutely, although it is usually has a more insidious onset. Symptoms will vary depending on the severity, but can be very debilitating.

The causes vary, but are usually associated with significant weight loss. It is often diagnosed late, and can require multiple investigations to confirm the diagnosis. Treatment is primarily aimed at increasing weight, but surgical intervention is often required.

We discuss the presentation and diagnosis of this rare condition, and treatment options.

INTRODUCTION

Superior mesenteric artery (SMA) syndrome is a rare clinical entity. It can have either an acute or chronic presentation, but the characteristic features of intermittent vomiting, fullness or satiety, and post prandial pain are common to both. It was first described in 1861 by the Austrian physician and philosopher Carl von Rokitansky [1], and since then has been recognised as being notoriously difficult to diagnose. As a result, it is a diagnosis frequently made by exclusion.

It is a high mechanical intestinal obstruction caused by partial or total obstruction of the third part of the duodenum where it passes between the superior mesenteric artery and posterior structures such as the aorta and vertebral column. This is due to loss of the mesenteric fat pad. The causes vary, but are usually associated with significant weight loss. Extensive investigations usually include an upper gastrointestinal contrast study, endoscopy, abdominal ultrasound (U/S), angiography and computer tomography.

It is often diagnosed late, and can require multiple investigations to confirm the diagnosis. Treatment is primarily aimed at increasing weight, and conservative medical management is advocated as the first line of treatment. However, surgical management is considered in cases where this has failed. Surgical approaches have evolved as advances in minimally invasive surgery have progressed.

The aim of this chapter is to discuss the pathophysiology, presentation and diagnosis of this condition, as well as treatment options available.

ANATOMY

The duodenum is the most proximal part of the small intestine. Its name originates from the Latin "*duodenum digitorum*" which translates to twelve fingers, reference to its length of approximately 12 fingers' breadth. Anatomically, the duodenum commences at the pylorus of the stomach and ends at the duodenojejunal junction. It is divided into four parts: these are termed first, second, third and fourth, or D1 to D4 respectively. Together the four parts wrap around the head of the pancreas to form a "C" shape. The superior portion of the duodenum exists at the spinal level L1 and is also known as "the cap." From the pylorus of the stomach, it ascends upwards, where the hepatoduodenal ligament adheres it to the liver. The proximal 2-3cm of D1 has an anterior and posterior covering of visceral peritoneum, whilst the remainder of the duodenum is a retroperitoneal structure, with a single anterior covering of peritoneum. The second part of the duodenum takes a descending path, curving inferiorly around the head of the pancreas. It lies from the spinal vertebral level of L1 through to L3, anterior to the right kidney and just posterior to the transverse colon. The portion of the Duodenum that undergoes compression in superior mesenteric artery syndrome is the third part. At the level of the L3 spinal vertebra, D3 travels to the left, and by doing so crosses the inferior vena cava and the aorta. It sits inferiorly to the uncinate process of the pancreas and posterior to the superior mesenteric vein and artery, the vascular bundle being responsible for causing the extrinsic compression of the duodenum in SMAS. Just after the duodenum has traversed the aorta at its lateral edge, it ascends sharply and curves anteriorly to join to the jejunum, the second part of the small bowel. This point is known as the duodenojejunal or DJ flexure.

Originating at the level of the first lumbar vertebrae on the anterior surface of the aorta, the superior mesenteric artery is the second major branch of the aorta in its abdominal portion. It originates, usually, between 0.5 cm and 1.5 cm inferior to the coeliac trunk, which is the artery that supplies the majority of embryonic foregut (stomach, spleen, pancreas and liver), and approximately the same distance superior to the renal arteries. Behind, or posterior to the artery, lies D3, together with the left renal vein and the pancreas. The left renal vein is nestled directly between the aorta and the origin of the SMA, which gives the propensity for obstruction of the said vein in certain circumstances. This obstruction is termed "nutcracker syndrome" which is discussed later in the chapter. The SMA provides blood supply to the third and fourth portions of the duodenum, plus all the jejunum and the ileum, and the first portion of the large bowel, specifically the caecum, ascending colon and the proximal portion of the transverse colon.

This corresponds to the embryological mid-gut. This commences in the distal or ampullary region of the second portion of the duodenum, right up to the splenic flexure of the colon. The descending and sigmoid colon take bloods supply from the inferior mesenteric artery, which is part of the embryological hindgut [2].

EARLY REPORTS

Superior mesenteric artery syndrome is a rare clinical entity, with a prevalence estimated between 0.0024-0.3% [1-3]. The first description was made by the Austrian professor Carl von Rokitansky in his principal work, the pathological anatomy textbook first published in 1842 [1]. Rokitansky was born in February 1804 in Bohemia and he attained a doctorate of medicine from the University of Vienna in 1828, at the age of 24. He recognised the relatively little known discipline of that time, namely pathological anatomy. He understood that this field could be of great importance, particularly in offering novel diagnostic and therapeutic possibilities to the bedside physician. As well as the first description of superior mesenteric artery syndrome, he also was the first to describe endometriosis in 1860 [3].

There were several case series of superior mesenteric artery syndrome published following Rokitansky's description [4]. However, it wasn't until Wilkie published the most comprehensive series of patients in 1922 that it became more recognised, and ever since his name has become an eponym for the syndrome. He describes the condition, initially it its grossest form, with the case of a 54-year-old female patient on whom he operated in the Royal Infirmary in Edinburgh, Scotland. This lady presented with symptoms of flatulent dyspepsia and vomiting. Unfortunately, she died as a result of duodenal ileus as a result of the extrinsic compression of the third part of the duodenum by the superior mesenteric vessels. There is also a second fatality described, as a young man with repeated and unrelenting bilious vomiting. By the time the patient was seen by Wilkie, he was in a particularly moribund condition, and died whilst his abdomen was being opened.

Writing more generally about the condition, Wilkie describes a typical patient with superior mesenteric artery syndrome as usually female, and often complaining of flatulent dyspepsia, pain or discomfort in the epigastrium, which commences between 30 and 120 minutes following a meal. Associated with these symptoms are feelings of distension "so pronounced that she may have to loosen her clothes to get ease." He goes on to describe other, less specific symptoms such as headaches, nausea, a loss of appetite and constipation and comments that attacks of vomiting are common, and often provide temporary relief to the symptoms. On the occasion where pain is a prominent feature of the presentation, he speculated on a proposed pathophysiology: a tonic pylorus resisting the regurgitation of the contents of the distended, obstructed duodenum back into the stomach, and hence increasing the pressure within the lumen of the duodenum; in turn this creating a greater stretch on the wall of the duodenum. When the pylorus relaxes, the reflux of the duodenal contents is allowed back into the stomach and hence the symptoms of pain subside. He went on to describe how several of his patients volunteered to him, that to lessen the symptoms and obtain some relief, they would lay on their face or adopt the genu-pectoral position. The mainstay of the treatment at the time of his writing was a duodenojejunostomy – this is an operation performed through a midline laparotomy incision, and where a portion of the mid small bowel, or the jejunum, is anastamosed or joined to the third part of the duodenum, just before the obstruction. At the time of writing, Wilkie had performed 21 cases, with uniform success, rapid improvement in symptoms and usually uninterrupted progress and weight gain.

The nomenclature of the syndrome has been varied over the years and includes: the aforesaid Wilkie's syndrome, arteriomesenteric duodenal compression, duodenal vascular compression and Cast syndrome [5]. Interestingly, Nutcracker syndrome is often mistakenly referred to at superior mesenteric artery syndrome but, although resulting from a very similar pathology, nutcracker syndrome refers to compression of the left renal vein by the SMA, not the duodenum.

It is now recognised that the underlying pathophysiology in the development of SMAS is due to loss of the mesenteric fat pad which allows the SMA 'drop down' towards the aorta. Several risk factors have been reported in the literature including anatomically altering surgery such as spinal scoliosis surgery where the spine is elongated, or panproctocolectomy and formation of ileoanal pouch for ulcerative colitis. Another broad group of risk factors for superior mesenteric artery syndrome are congenital abnormalities, broadly: malrotation, high insertion of the ligament of Treitz and a low origin of the SMA. The most common theme in the reports is that significant weight loss plays a role, and is another reported risk factor for superior mesenteric artery syndrome. This can encompass bariatric surgery, and eating disorders such as anorexia nervosa. Cast syndrome also has its basis is weight loss, due to long periods of time immobilised, reduced oral intake primarily due to restriction, resulted in wasting, and loss of the mesenteric fat pad. Following spinal cord injury, Christopher Reeve, BAFTA award winning actor for his role as the DC comic superhero Superman, suffered from acute superior mesenteric artery syndrome. However, despite the aforementioned risk factors being recognised, Akin et al. reported that in over 40% of cases there is no overt cause identified [6].

PRESENTATION AND DIAGNOSIS

The diagnosis of superior mesenteric artery syndrome is often challenging and usually only considered after the exclusion of a wide differential. Motility disorders and pancreatitis are key differentials to exclude, and it is also important to consider gastroesophageal reflux disease, biliary colic, mesenteric angina and peptic and duodenal ulcer disease [7]. The predominant clinical presentation encompasses often vague chronic upper abdominal symptoms, for example nausea and vomiting, epigastric pain (usually post prandial) and bloating. Weight loss is another key feature of the presentation; however this can be both a cause of the symptoms, as well as a consequence due to reduced oral intake.

Once the diagnosis is clinically suspected, the gold standard investigation is a barium swallow together with CT or MR angiography. It must be made clear however that because the clinical and the radiological findings are often transitory, diagnosis can easily overlooked if the history and investigations are taken and/or performed between discernible periods.

Computed tomography (CT) criteria for the diagnosis of SMA syndrome include an aortomesenteric angle of less than 22° and an aortomesenteric distance of less than 10mm. The aortomesenteric angle is formed between the aorta and the superior mesenteric artery at the point it crosses the third part of the duodenum, and the aortomesenteric distance is the distance between the aorta and the superior mesenteric artery in the inferior border of the third part of the duodenum (see Figure 1).

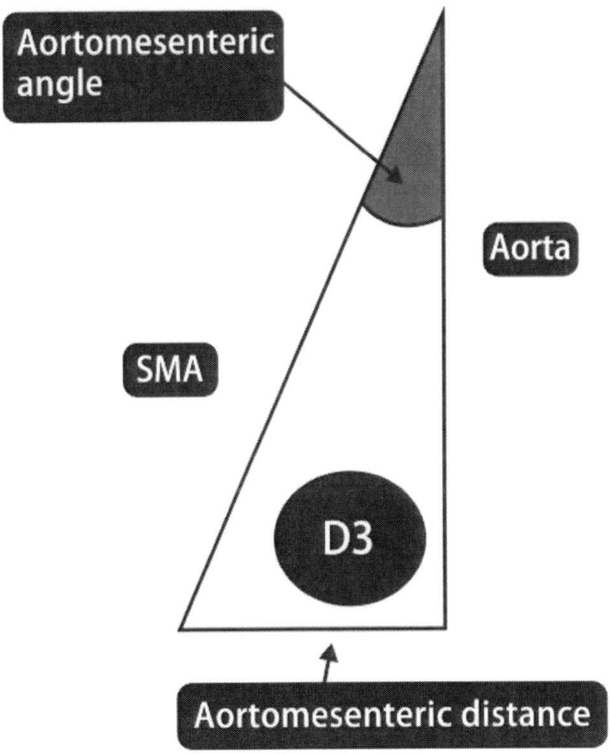

Figure 1. Defining the aortomesenteric angle

Within a healthy population of adults, the normal angle formed between the aorta and SMA is said to be 45° with a range of 25 to 60° [8]. In the normal population, there is strong correlation between these two measurements against BMI [9]. Other features of the diagnosis on CT include dilatation of the stomach and proximal transition point at point at which the SMA crosses the third part of the duodenum [10]. Upper GI endoscopy may reveal a pulsatile extrinsic compression of the duodenum in its third portion.

Several studies looking at upper gastrointestinal barium examinations in patients with superior mesenteric artery syndrome found the important diagnostic criteria to be duodenal dilatation combined with an indentation in the duodenum caused by the SMA [8]. However, Lukes et al. suggested that duodenal dilatation may not always be shown. [11] Forwards and backwards movement, indicating antiperastalsis or the result of forward movement against a blockage, was also found to be highly significant when achieving the correct diagnosis [12, 13]. Birsen et al. reported CT findings of patients with superior mesenteric artery syndrome where gastric dilatation and a reduced aorto-SMA distance was present in all subjects, and that there was close correlation demonstrated between clinical findings or suspected diagnosis, and the radiological findings. Gastric dilatation was deemed to be when the presence of gastric rugal flattening with circumferential gastric wall thinning was combined with large air-fluid levels. They proposed that the aforesaid two CT findings should create a suspicion of the pathology, even if not all diagnostic criteria are met [8].

Prognosis and Complications

The prognosis and incidence of complications of SMA syndrome is frequently related to the delay in achieving the correct diagnosis. Often, the delay in diagnosis is associated with poorer outcomes, and can result in a wide ranging collection of complications including: dehydration and electrolyte abnormalities, renal failure, malnutrition, gastritis and oesophagitis, GI haemorrhage, gastric perforation, aspiration pneumonia and death. There has been a reported association of 25-45% with peptic ulcer disease and up to 50% with hyperchlorhydria [14].

Treatment

Due to the often-delayed diagnosis, treatment in the first instance tends to be related to resolving the complications of the condition, such as correction of electrolyte imbalances, intravenous hydration and amendment of renal failure and decompression of a distended stomach via an NG tube. Mobilisation into the prone or left lateral decubitus position often is helpful in an acute setting [15]. Other conservative management approaches that have suggested to be of help include parenteral nutrition, nasojejunal tube feeding which bypasses the point of obstruction, and input of a dietician. Metoclopromide as well as other pro-kinetic agents have been found to be useful in some cases, particularly when the obstruction is partial.

Failure of conservative treatments may result in the necessity of surgery. However, it has been proposed that conservative management should usually be tried for a minimum period of 6 weeks to 3 months prior to considering surgery. Major advancements in nutrition in the last few decades have resulted in a substantial shift away from surgical treatment towards medical treatment. Two paediatric cohorts were compared from 1974 and 2006, and the need for surgical treatment had reduced from 70% to 14% [14].

Surgical Treatment

The surgical options for the treatment of superior mesenteric artery syndrome all aim to address the obstruction by bypassing the obstructed segment. There are three mainstay options, which include: duodenojejunostomy, gastrojejunostomy and division of the ligament of Treitz with de-rotation of the bowel (Strong's procedure).

The first reported duodenojejunostomy for superior mesenteric artery syndrome was performed by Stavely in 1908, and this has become the most frequent and successful procedure reported in the literature, with a success rate approaching 80% [16]. From a review by Lee and Mangla in 1978, it was concluded that from 1963, 146 cases were reviewed, and duodenojejunostomy revealed the best results in severe cases, and that it was superior in results to both gastrojejunostomy and Strong's procedure [17].

With the advent of minimally invasive, or keyhole surgery, so came the laparoscopic approach to the treatment of superior mesenteric artery syndrome. The first to describe the laparoscopic duodenojejunostomy to treat superior mesenteric artery syndrome were Gersin and Heniford in 1998, at the Cleveland Clinic, Ohio, USA [18]. They performed this first on a 24 year old female with a previous history of abdominal colectomy and ileorectal anastamosis, who had failed conservative management. There have been subsequent reports from Richardson and Surowiec, Kim et al. Bermas and Fenoglio and Kingham et al. that have collectively concluded that laparoscopic management is a safe alternative to the open approach, with added superiorities in a reduced procedure time and reduced time of recovery [19-22].

Wyten et al. described a case series of laparoscopic duodenojejunostomy for the treatment of superior mesenteric artery syndrome including the case of a 41-year-old female presenting with an acute history of right upper quadrant pain. She had further associated symptoms that included a fever, nausea and vomiting. Her past medical history included quadriplegia as a result of a C6-C7 subluxation, cervical myelopathy, rheumatoid arthritis, psoriasis and a recent cholecystectomy 7 weeks previously. Serum liver function testing was abnormal, and given the recent surgical history, she was commenced on antibiotics as treatment for presumed cholangitis. An abdominal radiograph demonstrated a dilated stomach and proximal duodenum, which was decompressed with the insertion of a nasogastric tube. Abdominal ultrasound scan was unremarkable, and ensued five days of conservative management. There was little resolution to the patient's symptomology and hence a CT scan of the abdomen was performed. This demonstrated dilation of the stomach and proximal duodenum to the point that the duodenum passed between the aorta and SMA. A diagnosis of superior mesenteric artery syndrome was made. Following the diagnosis, there was a further attempt at a period of conservative management. Despite this, the patient failed to improve and she was taken to theatre for a laparoscopic duodenojejunostomy. The steps of the procedure are succinctly described as follows:

> "A capnoperitoneum was established via the insertion of a 10mm laparoscopic instrument port though an incision through the umbilicus. Three further 5mm ports were inserted into the abdomen. The omentum was dissected away from the second and third parts of the duodenum. Intraoperatively at this point, it was observed that the whole stomach, and first and second parts of the duodenum was grossly dilated, with associated small bowel collapsed distal to the duodenum. Stay sutures were placed to elevate the transverse colon and a window was identified and developed with electrocautery lateral to the middle colic vessels gaining exposure of the duodenum. The duodenum was mobilised using a partial kocherisation technique. A portion of the jejunum was juxtaposed to the duodenum and a stay suture placed. Enterotomies were made in both in both aforesaid loops of bowel. A 45 mm staple gun was inserted into and across the two enterotomies and a single fire was performed. The final enterotomy was closed again with a single fire of a staple gun. The stapled anastamosis was intact and the staple line was haemostatic… Following the procedure, the patient gained weight, and remained symptoms free up to and including a 2.5-year postoperative outpatient clinic visit, after which she was discharged." [23]

Further reported cases within the series ensued a similar course, with low operating times and quick postoperative recovery with cessation of pain. The series highlights that laparoscopic duodenojejunostomy is an appropriate form of surgical management in patients with superior mesenteric artery syndrome who have failed a conservative approach to management. The significant advantages of this approach over a traditional open operative approach results in both a shorter operating time, and length of recovery.

Another surgical approach widely reported is a gastrojejunostomy. This is where a loop of jejunum is brought up and anastomosed onto the stomach. This then in turn bypasses the duodenum where the point of obstruction is. Although adequate gastric decompression can be achieved from this technique, failure to deal with the duodenal obstruction can lead to persistence of symptoms and ultimately blind loop syndrome, resulting in gastric bile reflux and ulceration [24]. It furthermore can lead to bacterial overgrowth and the resultant bacteria cause breakdown of bile salts and deamination of some proteins. This in turn can lead to deficiencies in fat-soluble vitamins, malabsorption and steatorrhea [17].

In 1958, Edward K. Strong, a surgeon at the Southern Pacific Hospital, San Francisco, California described the mechanics of superior mesenteric artery syndrome and proposed a direct surgical approach to treatment. This is now what is commonly referred to as Strong's procedure. This was performed by division of the ligament of Trietz. First described by an Austrian physician Wenzel Treitz in 1853, this eponymous ligament is the suspensory ligament of the duodenum [25]. The ligament of Treitz lies posterior to the pancreas and anterior to the left renal vein. It is comprised of two parts: the upper part, also termed the Hilfsmuskel, arises at the oesophageal hiatus from the diaphragmatic crus. It consists of skeletal muscle, which becomes fibrous tissue in its distal portion, terminating with insertion into the celiac axis. The inferior part of the ligament is the suspensory muscle of the duodenum and this arises directly from the duodenum. Unlike the superior part, this is smooth muscle that becomes fibrous again in its distal portion and joins with the Hilfsmuskel in its insertion into the celiac axis. It is reported however that there is significant anatomical variation of these structures [26].

In his 1958 paper, Strong very eloquently describes superior mesenteric artery syndrome, and the biomechanics of the pathology:

> "In its transverse or ascending portion depending on individual variation, the duodenum usually lies in an acute vascular angle between the aorta and the superior mesenteric artery. If we could liken the superior mesenteric artery to a surveyor's plumb-line and the weight of the small bowel and its mesentery to the plumb-bob, then the superior mesenteric artery-aortic angle would approach 90 degrees in the quadruped and less than 0 degrees in the human with normal lumbar lordosis. Obviously evolution would have stopped short of the biped human if erect posture in itself resulted in duodenal obstruction." [27]

Strong introduces his procedure in the format of a case report of a 30 year old male yardman, who is saw in October 1956 with symptoms of weight loss of 30lbs within one year, indigestion and abdominal pains for 1 year's duration. Radiological examinations confirmed a large stomach, and enlarged first and second parts of the duodenum. At this time, Strong made the diagnosis of "*chronic duodenal stasis secondary to compression of the duodenum by the superior mesenteric artery.*" Strong took the patient to the operating theatre and performed a laparotomy, where the findings mirrored the radiological evidence gathered. The gastric pylorus was said to be distended to 4-5cm, and the duodenum distended to the point at which the superior mesenteric artery crossed it. There was an indentation found in the anterior aspect of the third part of the duodenum caused by the evidently obstructing superior mesenteric artery. The duodenum in its distal portion after the presumed point of obstruction was of normal calibre. The procedure is described in a stepwise manner with the Trietz ligament being divided initially, followed by delicate stripping of the duodenum across its avascular plane between the superior surface of the duodenum and the inferior surface of the pancreas. Whilst the pancreas remained a retroperitoneal structure, the fourth part of the duodenum was transformed into an "intraperitoneal" structure. The procedure resulted in rapid reversal of symptomology and of radiological evidence of obstruction in the presented case.

CONCLUSION

Superior mesenteric artery syndrome was first described in the mid 19th century at autopsy, however as a clinically relevant pathology, it remained absent from literature until Wilkie published the first series in 1922. It remains a very rare entity, with a vague, non-specific presentation which results in a frequently difficult and controversial diagnosis. This is in part due to the confusion and crossover with a number of different (and more common) conditions [28]. However it is a recognised clinical entity, and the longer taken to make the diagnosis can result in significant morbidity [29].

Due to the lack of specific features, the chronicity and weight loss should result in clinical suspicion that can lead to inclusion of superior mesenteric artery syndrome within a differential. The gold standard investigations are barium contrast study of the upper GI tract, and CT of the abdomen with calculation of the SMA angle and distance.

The mainstay of treatment is non-surgical to address weight loss and the complications of the condition. This has been helped by the significant improvements in nutritional sciences and parenteral nutrition. However, surgical intervention has been shown to be highly effective with minimal associated morbidity in patients who fail conservative management.

REFERENCES

[1] Rokitansky, K., *Handbuch der pathologischen anatomie*.[Manual of pathological anatomy] Vol. 3. 1842: Vienna : Braumuller & Seidel.

[2] Shaikh, H. and A. Khorasani-Zadeh, *Anatomy, Abdomen and Pelvis, Superior Mesenteric Artery*, in *StatPearls*. 2018: Treasure Island (FL).

[3] Benagiano, G., I. Brosens, and D. Lippi, *The History of Endometriosis*. Vol. 78. 2014.

[4] Laffer, W. B., *VI.* Acute Dilatation of the Stomach and Arterio-Mesenteric Ileus. *Ann Surg,* 1908. 47(3): p. 390-416.

[5] Zaraket, V. and L. Deeb, Wilkie's Syndrome or Superior Mesenteric Artery Syndrome: Fact or Fantasy? *Case Rep Gastroenterol*, 2015. 9(2): p. 194-9.

[6] Akin, J. T., Jr., S. W. Gray, and J. E. Skandalakis, Vascular compression of the duodenum: Presentation of ten cases and review of the literature. *Surgery*, 1976. 79(5): p. 515-22.

[7] Merrett, N. D., et al. Superior mesenteric artery syndrome: diagnosis and treatment strategies. *J Gastrointest Surg*, 2009. 13(2): p. 287-92.

[8] Unal, B., et al. Superior mesenteric artery syndrome: CT and ultrasonography findings. *Diagn Interv Radiol*, 2005. 11(2): p. 90-5.

[9] Ozkurt, H., et al. Measurement of the distance and angle between the aorta and superior mesenteric artery: normal values in different BMI categories. *Surg Radiol Anat*, 2007. 29(7): p. 595-9.

[10] Biswas, A., et al. Superior mesenteric artery syndrome: CT findings. *BMJ Case Rep*, 2016. 2016.

[11] Lukes, P. J., et al. Diagnostic value of hypotonic duodenography in superior mesenteric artery syndrome. *Acta Chir Scand*, 1978. 144(1): p. 39-43.

[12] Rosa-Jimenez, F., et al. Duodenal compression caused by superior mesenteric artery: study of 10 patients. *Rev Esp Enferm Dig*, 2003. 95(7): p. 485-9, 480-4.

[13] Hines, J. R., R. M. Gore, and G. H. Ballantyne, Superior mesenteric artery syndrome. Diagnostic criteria and therapeutic approaches. *Am J Surg*, 1984. 148(5): p. 630-2.

[14] Biank, V. and S. Werlin, Superior mesenteric artery syndrome in children: a 20-year experience. *J Pediatr Gastroenterol Nutr*, 2006. 42(5): p. 522-5.

[15] Dietz, U. A., et al. [*Aorto-mesenteric artery compression syndrome*]. Chirurg [Surgeon], 2000. 71(11): p. 1345-51.

[16] Lundell, L. and A. Thulin, Wilkie's syndrome--a rarity? *Br J Surg*, 1980. 67(8): p. 604-6.

[17] Lee, C. S. and J. C. Mangla, Superior mesenteric artery compression syndrome. *Am J Gastroenterol*, 1978. 70(2): p. 141-50.

[18] Gersin, K. S. and B. T. Heniford, Laparoscopic duodenojejunostomy for treatment of superior mesenteric artery syndrome. *JSLS,* 1998. **2**(3): p. 281-4.

[19] Richardson, W. S. and W. J. Surowiec, Laparoscopic repair of superior mesenteric artery syndrome. *Am J Surg,* 2001. 181(4): p. 377-8.

[20] Kim, I. Y., et al. Laparoscopic duodenojejunostomy for management of superior mesenteric artery syndrome: two cases report and a review of the literature. *Yonsei Med J,* 2003. 44(3): p. 526-9.

[21] Bermas, H. and M. E. Fenoglio, Laparoscopic management of superior mesenteric artery syndrome. *JSLS*, 2003. **7**(2): p. 151-3.

[22] Kingham, T. P., R. Shen, and C. Ren, Laparoscopic treatment of superior mesenteric artery syndrome. *JSLS*, 2004. 8(4): p. 376-9.

[23] Wyten, R., C. J. Kelty, and G. L. Falk, Laparoscopic duodenojejunostomy for the treatment of superior mesenteric artery (SMA) Syndrome: case series. *J Laparoendosc Adv Surg Tech A*, 2010. 20(2): p. 173-6.

[24] Stewart, B. A., et al. The blind loop syndrome in children. *J Pediatr Surg*, 1990. 25(8): p. 905-8.

[25] Treitz, W., Uber Einen Neven Muskel Am Duodenum. *Vjschr prakt Heilk,* 1853. 37: p. 113-144.

[26] Kim, S .K., C. D. Cho, and A. R. Wojtowycz, The ligament of Treitz (the suspensory ligament of the duodenum): anatomic and radiographic correlation. *Abdom Imaging,* 2008. 33(4): p. 395-7.

[27] Strong, E. K., Mechanics of arteriomesentric duodenal obstruction and direct surgical attack upon etiology. *Ann Surg,* 1958. 148(5): p. 725-30.

[28] Cohen, L. B., S. P. Field, and D. B. Sachar, The superior mesenteric artery syndrome. The disease that isn't, or is it? *J Clin Gastroenterol,* 1985. **7**(2): p. 113-6.

[29] Shetty, A. K., et al. Radiological case of the month. Superior mesenteric artery syndrome. *Arch Pediatr Adolesc Med*, 1999. 153(3): p. 303-4.

In: Horizons in World Cardiovascular … ISBN: 978-1-53616-157-1
Editor: Eleanor H. Bennington

Chapter 4

SURGICAL ANATOMY OF THE SUPERIOR MESENTERIC ARTERY

Antonio Manenti[1,*], Gabriele Melegari[1], Alberto Farinetti[1] and Gianrocco Manco[1]
[1]Department of Surgery, University of Modena, Modena, Italy

ABSTRACT

The superior mesenteric artery (SMA) can be subdivided into three segments for an easier comprehension of its surgical anatomy.

The first segment is the most proximally placed, behind the body of the pancreas; the second is positioned medially to the duodeno-jejunal junction, and the third, the most distal, is located at the base of mesenteries of the transverse colon and of the small bowel. This spatial arrangement involves different surgical approaches.

The dissection of the first segment is the most challenging and requires a surgical approach through the retroperitoneum, medially displacing the left colon and the spleno-pancreatic block. The second segment is approached by mobilizing the duodeno-jejunal junction, and the third, through dissecting at the base of the mesenteries of the transverse colon and of the small bowel.

[*] Corresponding Author's Email: antonio.manenti@unimore.it.

In case of pancreatic cancer, a secondary involvement of the SMA can be verified through its direct exploration, performed with a Kocher's maneuver in cephalic tumors, or moving down the duodeno-jejunal junction in tumors of the body or of the tail of the pancreas.

INTRODUCTION

For a better understanding, the surgical anatomy of the superior mesenteric artery (SMA) can be simply schematized through a subdivision in three segments, each with a different method for surgical dissection [1, 2].

1) The first segment is located just downstream of its origin behind the pancreatic body.
2) The second segment continues crossing the third part of the duodenum, above the left renal vein.
3) The third segment, the infra-mesocolic, crosses the base of the transverse colon mesentery and runs inside the ileum.

In any case, the choice among the different approaches to SMA is based on a previous accurate imaging study, essential for a precise clinical diagnosis [3]. In open surgery, the median laparotomy remains the preferred way, suitable for all the three segments.

ANATOMO-SURGICAL DETAILS

Surgical dissection of the *SMA 1st segment* continues to be challenging, being completely placed in a retro-pancreatic space. It requires a large exposition, usually performed by the Mattox's maneuver: it consists of a medial mobilization of the left colon, together with the spleno-pancreatic block. The retroperitoneal space is approached, leaving the left adrenal gland, the left kidney surrounded by the Gerota fascia and the left renal vein behind . This maneuver exposes the abdominal aorta from the celiac trunk to the inferior mesenteric artery, together with its other collaterals, the SMA, and the left renal artery. At the same time, the left renal vein is dissected (Figure 1).

The surgical approach to the other SMA segments is realized in the infra-meso-colic space, reached by lifting up the transvers colon and the greater omentum.

In particular, the *SMA 2nd segment*, the juxta-duodenal, is approached dividing the Treitz's ligament and dislocating the duodeno-jejunal junction down and medially (Figure 2) [4].

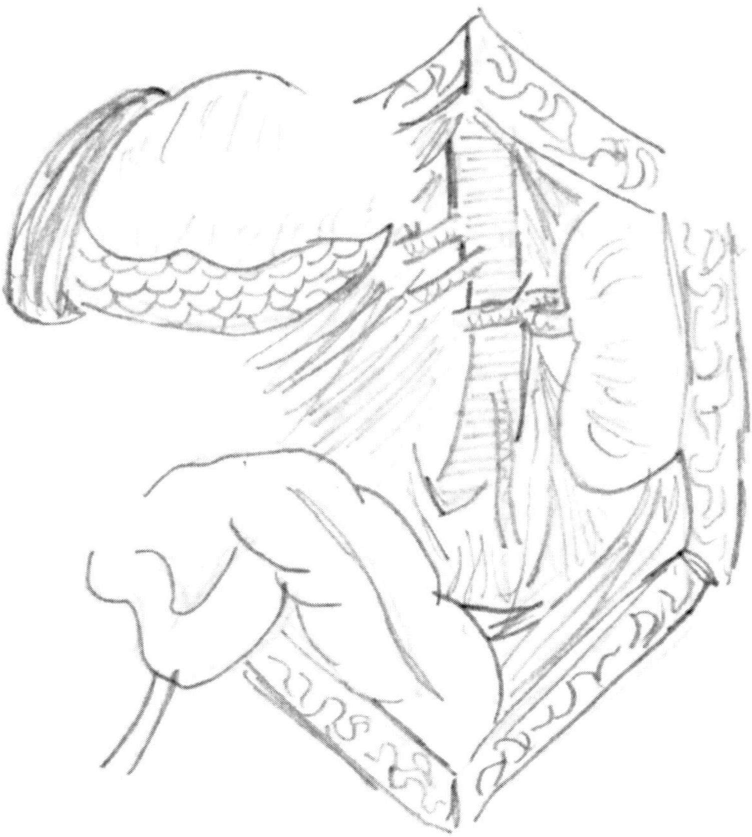

Figure 1. Mattox's maneuver to dissect the SMA 1st segment.

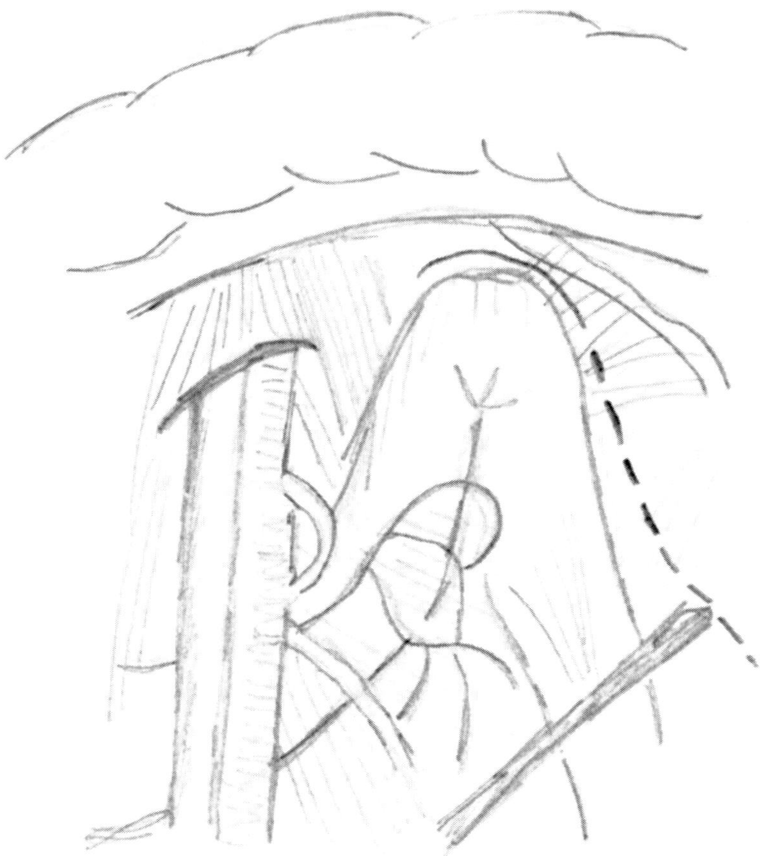

Figure 2. The SMA 2nd segment is approached in the infra-mesocolic space dividing the Treitz's ligament and displacing down and medially the duodeno-jejunal junction. The inferior mesenteric vein is preserved.

This SMA segment is found between the aorta and the inferior mesenteric vein, wrapped by many vegetative nervous fibers. Its collaterals are represented by branches to the first jejunal loop and by the pancreato-duodenal vessels that must be preserved. At the back of this plane, the left renal vein can be easily exposed. The inferior mesenteric vein, which runs laterally, can be divided to enlarge the space of dissection.

The *SMA 3rd segment* allows an easier and more direct approach. It is performed always in the infra-mesocolic space, lifting up the transverse colon, extending its mesentery, and displacing the first jejunal loop laterally (Figure 3). At the base of the small bowel mesentery, on the left side of the aorta, the SMA can be felt as a pulsating structure or as a stretched cord. This approach allows to lengthen the dissection more distally, to expose the SMA right branches until the ileo-caeco-colic artery; as a rule, these branches, are to be saved (1).

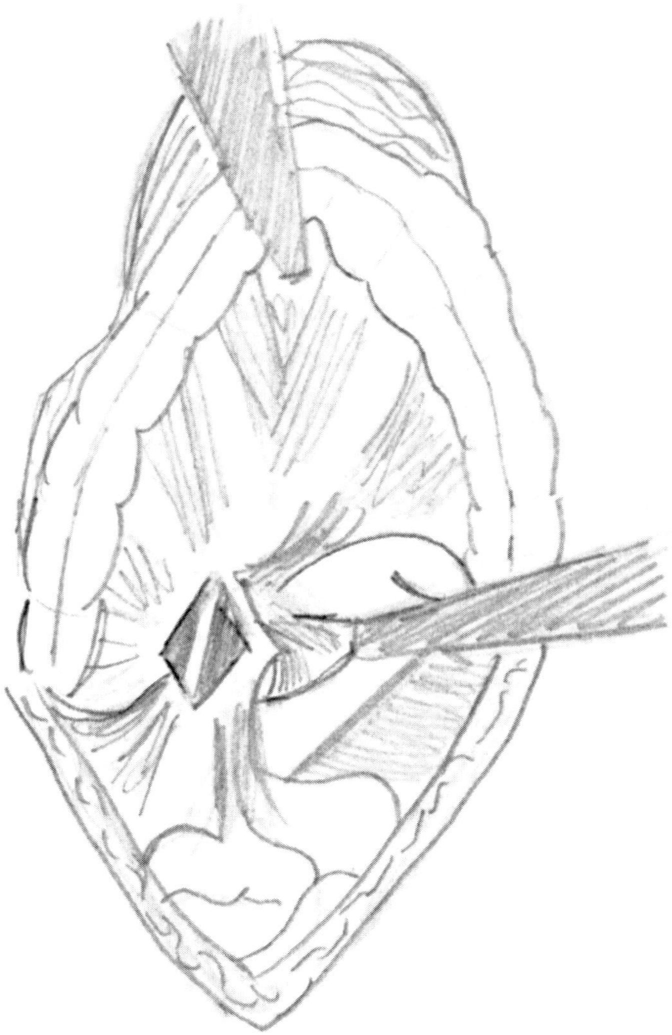

Figure 3. The SMA 3rd segment is dissected along the mesentery root.

Interestingly, this tract of the SMA, downstream of the middle colic branch, represents the elective site of embolization. This dissection allows a hybrid surgical-radiological procedure, consisting in a retrograde SMA catheterization and stenting, in order to resolve proximal obstructions [5].

Clearly, this approach, the most direct, can be proposed such as the first surgical step, foregoing and facilitating dissection of the second segment: so a larger SMA exposition is reached.

ACUTE SURGICAL CONDITIONS

All these methods of dissection are already proposed in cases of SMA chronic vascular diseases, and can be applied also in emergency conditions, such as embolization or acute thrombosis. However, they demand a careful and complete exploration of all the intestinal loops, to detect segments of frank or sub-critical ischemia.

ONCOLOGICAL CONDITIONS

In pancreatic cancer surgery, the dissection of the SMA, mainly in its retro-pancreatic segment, is suggested to control intra-operatively its secondary involvement. This represents a first exploratory step of pancreatectomy.

In particular, in surgery of pancreatic head cancer, the first SMA segment can be explored with a Kocher's maneuver, extended until the anterior wall of the aorta. In this way, the SMA first segment, in its complete retro-pancreatic tract, is exposed downstream to its origin [6-9].

This oncological surgery often requires the exploration of the superior mesenteric vein: a Cattell-Braasch maneuver enables the contemporary exploration of the SMA second segment.

When a duodeno-pancreatectomy is extended to include resection of the corresponding SMA retro-pancreatic segment, the subsequent arterial reconstruction can be performed through an interposed graft or, more simply, with a direct re-implantation of the distal SMA stump in the infra-renal aorta [11].

In case of a distal spleno-pancreatectomy for tumors of the pancreatic tail, the SMA can be explored in its second segment, as described above, dividing the Treitz's ligament and displacing the duodeno-jejunal junction down and medially.

References

[1] Shaikh, H. and Bhimji, S. S. (2018) *Anatomy, abdomen and pelvis, superior mesenteric artery*. Stat. Pearls Publishing, 2018-Sept. 13.

[2] Alsabilah, J., Kim, W. R. and Kim, N. K. (2017) Vascular structures of the right colon: incidence and variations with their clinical implications. *Scand. J. Surg.,* 106 (2), 107 - 115.

[3] Wilkins, L. R. and Stone, R. (2015) Chronic mesenteric ischemia. *Tech. Vasc. Interv. Radiol.,* 18 (1), 24 - 30.

[4] Al-Asari, S. F., Lim, D., Min, B. S. and Kim, N. K. (2013) The relation between inferior mesenteric vein ligation and collateral vessels to splenic flexure: anatomical landmarks, technical precautions and clinical significance. *Yonsei Med. J.,* 54 (6), 1484 - 1490.

[5] Oderich, G. S., Macedo, R., Ston, D. H., Woo, E. Y., Panneton, J. M., Resch, T. et al. (2018) Multicentric study for retrograde open mesenteric artery stenting through laparotomy for treatment of acute and chronic mesenteric ischemia. *J. Vasc. Surg.,* 68, (2), 470 - 480.

[6] Pessaux, P., Rosso, E., Panaro, F., Marzano, E., Oussoultzoglou, E., Bachellier, P. et al. (2009) Preliminary experience with the hanging maneuver for pancreaticoduodenectomy. *Eur. J. Surg. Oncol.,* 35 (9), 1006 - 1010.

[7] Weitz, J., Rahbari, N., Koch, M. and Büchler, M. W. (2010) The "artery first" approach for resection of pancreatic head cancer. *J. Am. Coll. Surg.,* 210 (2), e1-4.

[8] Inoue, Y., Saiura, A., Tanaka, M., Matsumura, M., Takeda, Y., Mise, Y. et al. (2016) Technical details of an anterior Approach to the

superior mesenteric artery during pancreaticoduodenectomy. *J. Gastrointest. Surg.*, 20(10):1769 - 1777.

[9] Aosasa, S., Nishikawa, M., Hoshikawa, M., Noro, T. and Yamamoto, J. (2016) Inframesocolic superior mesenteric artery first approach as an introductory procedure of radical antegrade modular pancreatosplenectomy for carcinoma of the pancreatic body and tail. *J. Gastrointest. Surg.*, 20(2):450 - 4.

[10] Del Chiaro, M., Segersvärd, R., Rangelova, E., Coppola, A., Scandavini, C. M., Ansorge, C. et al. (2015) Cattell-Braasch maneuver combined with artery-first approach for superior mesenteric-portal vein resection during pancreatectomy. *J. Gastrointest. Surg.*, 19 (12):2264 - 2268.

[11] Manenti, A., Melegari, G., Manco, G. and Farinetti, A. (2018) Re-implanting the superior mesenteric artery on the infra-renal aorta. *Surgery*, 163 (4), 970.

In: Horizons in World Cardiovascular ... ISBN: 978-1-53616-157-1
Editor: Eleanor H. Bennington

Chapter 5

ZEBRAFISH MODELS FOR SCREENING OF CARDIOTOXIC AGENTS AND IT EXISTS OUTSIDE THE AMBIT OF CARDIOVASCULAR RESEARCH

Arunachalam Muthuraman*, Rajavel Varatharajan and K. Jaya Raja Kumar
Pharamacology Unit, Faculty of Pharmacy, AIMST University, Semeling, Bedong, Kedah Darul Aman, Malaysia

ABSTRACT

Over the past decade, zebrafishes have been employed as a key model for various drug screening processes such as cancer, infectious disease, neurodegeneration, pain, dementia, toxicology and so on. This chapter focused on the current development of zebrafish models for the screening for cardiotoxic and cardioprotective agents. Various methods have been employed in the development of cardiotoxicity in zebrafish. The administration or exposure of endocrine disruptors, cigarette smoke, acrylamide, phthalates & phosphate, heavy metals, inoculation infectious agent, alcohol, surgery (cryosection & amputation) and laser light radiations are the major cause of cardiotoxicity in zebrafish. Hence,

* Corresponding Author's Email: arunachalammu@gmail.com.

zebrafishes have been considered as an appropriate tool in the assessment of cardiotoxicity in experimental research and drug discovery process due to numerous advantages over mammalian models. Further, it allows analyzing the variety of cardiovascular and hemodynamic parameters. Therefore, zebrafish can broaden horizons in the field of cardiovascular research.

Keywords: cardiotoxicity, *Danio rerio*, degeneration, drug screening, endocrine disruptors, zebrafish embryo

ABBREVIATIONS

AA,	acrylic amide;
ACR,	acrylamide;
ACTC,	Alpha cardiac actin;
BA,	bulbus arteriosus;
BBP,	butyl benzyl phthalate;
BPA,	bisphenol-A;
BPAF,	bisphenol AF;
BPB,	bisphenol B;
BPF,	bisphenol F;
BPS,	bisphenol S;
CHD,	congenital heart diseases;
CM,	cardiomyocyte;
CPCs,	cardiac progenitor cells;
CS,	cigarette smoke;
CVDs,	cardiovascular disorders;
DA,	diterpene alkaloids;
DAU,	daunorubicin;
DBP,	dibutyl phthalate;
dpa,	days post-amputation;
dpf,	days post fertilization;
ECG,	electrocardiogram;
EF,	ejection fraction;
EGFP,	enhanced green fluorescent protein;

FLK1,	vascular endothelial growth factor (VEGF);
GATA4,	erythroid transcription factor;
GATA4/5/6,	GATA erythroid transcription factor;
HAND2,	Helix-loop-helix transcription factor;
hpf,	hours post fertilization;
hpi,	hours post injury;
KCNH2,	potassium channel, voltage gated eagrelated subfamily H, member 2;
MCSF,	macrophage colony-stimulating factor;
MYH6,	Alpha myosin heavy chain;
NKX2.5,	Homeobox containing transcription factor 2-5;
NOTCH1,	Notch homolog1;
P&P,	phthalatesand phosphate;
RA,	retinoic acid;
RAR,	retinoic acid receptor;
RXR,	retinoid receptors;
SEMA3,	Semaphorin 3;
SMAD,	human homologue of Mad and Sma proteins;
SMAD6,	SMAD family member 6;
SV,	sinus venosus;
T-box-5,	T-box transcription factor 5;
TITIN,	titin gene;
TPP,	triphenyl phosphate;
zfER,	zebrafish specific estrogen receptor;
and zfER-β_2,	zebrafish specific estrogen β_2 receptor.

INTRODUCTION

Globally cardiovascular disorders (CVD) are the leading cause of death. The occurrences of CVDs arise from birth to death at any age due to multiple etiological factors [1]. In the drug discovery process, the screenings of cardiovascular medicines are relying on animal models [2-3]. The various animal models are employed for the evaluation of lead molecule for the

CVD treatment. Moreover, the lead molecules are partially identified by *in-silico* molecular docking process via drug-protein interaction and testing on the cardiomyocytes [4-5]. However; exact toxicity, efficacy, potency and pharmacokinetic profiles including adverse drug reactions are evaluated in experimental animal models [6-7]. In research laboratories, there are some animals are engaged for the screening of novel lead molecule in various disorders; such animal species are rat, mice, rabbit, gerbil, and dogs [8-9]. However, the emerging field of cardiovascular research is needed for the development of more effective bioactive molecules. The identification of lead molecules for CVDs with conventional animal models is too expensive and time-consuming. Therefore, newer species are identified i.e., zebrafish (*Danio rerio*). It has a wide variety of advantage over the conventional mammalian animal species [2, 10].

The major advantages of the zebrafish model in cardiovascular research are structural and function genome data availability like human genome; easy to apply the gene knock-out and knock-in process; allowed to apply genetic engineering techniques; possible to edit the host gene; shorter generation time; high fecundity; external fertilization process; accessibility of developmental changes; transparency of embryo; possibility to make real-time imaging; and efficient absorption of small molecular weight compounds from water resources [11-14]. The additional advantages of zebrafish models are vertebrate, easy to maintain and inexpensive animal species [11, 15]. However, it also has some limitation such as prototypical heart not similar to the structure and functions like a mammalian heart; small size, so difficult to collect the complete physiological data; the development of heart-related behavior complication is lower; less reliable when using insoluble drugs [16-17]. Congenital heart diseases (CHDs) are one of the common variety of birth-related cardiac functional defect [18]. Further, it alters the cardiac output and clinical outcome is poor [19-20]. Hence, zebrafish models can be considered as one of the best models for the assessment of CHDs. In addition, various factors are employed in the progression of CVDs for screening newer cardiovascular acting agents in zebrafish models. Further, the maximal CVDs has been exposed in larvae stages of zebrafish [21-25]. However, some of the studies are also documented in adult zebrafish [18, 22, 25-26]. In addition, the route of cardio-toxin exposure is mainly via water source with soluble cardiotoxin. The developmental cardiotoxicity was observed from fertilized eggs i.e., 24 hours post fertilization (hpf) and it is also known as embryonic heart [27-28].

MORPHOGENESIS OF ZEBRAFISH HEART

The zebrafish heart has two chambers instead of four chambers of the mammalian heart. And, it has similar cellular and molecular strategies of the mammalian heart [12, 29]. Further, it allows the assessment of optical transparency with fluorescent markers labeled cardiac cells [30-31]. However, the major and important fact of zebrafish embryogenesis is not requiring a specific functional cardiovascular system in the first week of zebrafish life leads to the minimal requirement of oxygen supply to tissue growth process [2, 32-33]. Whereas, the heart is a first organ in the development of mammalian heart [34]. Thus, zebrafish helps to assess the clinical relevant CHDs. The contraction of zebrafish heart initiates from 24 hpf [35-36]. The developmental heart composed of three major cell types i.e., atrial cardiomyocytes (CM), ventricular CM, and endocardial cells [37]. Thus, differentiated cells i.e., cardiac progenitor cells (CPCs) can be traces at 5 hpf in the lateral marginal surface of blastula [38-39]. The migration of progenitor cells is observed during the gastrulation process in the posterior half of the anterior lateral plate of mesoderm at 15 hpf [40]. Followed by CPCs are fuse into endocardial cells which is recline in center of ventricular and atrial myocytes [41]. Crucially, the linear tube was extending with distinct protein expression for atrial CM, ventricular CM and endocardial cells [39]. At 48 hpf the looped heart is formed and it has a pericardial cavity and clear heart (two) chamber with atrio-ventricular blood flow [2, 42]. Even though, it is still considered as immature heart due to lack of auxiliary cell types and additional structural features of the heart for function i.e., bulbous arteriosus, valve cushions, valve leaflets, myocardial protrusions (trabeculae and epicardium) [10, 43]. Approximately at 72 hpf the myocardium expands and ready to spreads cardiac-resident cells like cardiac fibroblasts; which is helps to the formation of endocardial trabeculae [44]. At 40 hpf, atrio-ventricular CMs are undergone the epithelial-to-mesenchymal transition to make the endocardial cushion followed by generates the primitive valve leaflets for allowing unidirectional blood flow [45]. This process is complete at 76 hpf. Later, it withstands thicken and lengthens of the cardiac valve to become mature valve [2]. It is also known as valvulogenesis [46]. Final steps of cardiogenesis are the maturation of heart. The maturation of zebrafish cardiac chamber continues from juvenile to early adult stage of zebrafish life. The morphogenesis of the zebrafish heart at different stages is illustrated in Figure 1.

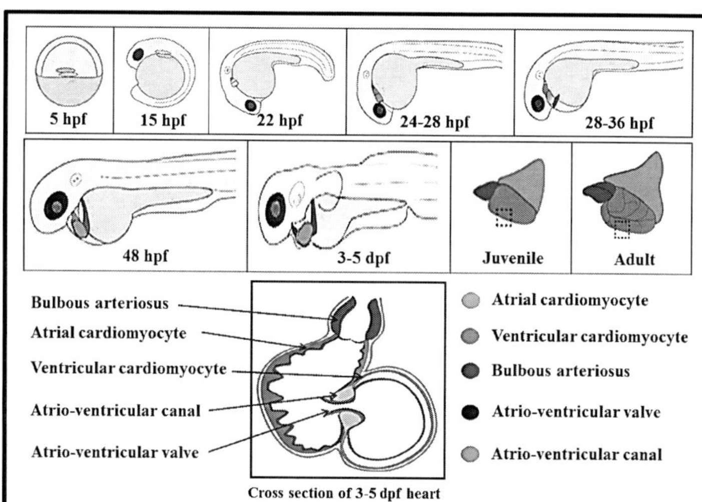

Abbreviations: hpf, hours post fertilization; dpf, days post fertilization.

Figure 1. Morphogenesis of zebrafish heart at different stages.

Phenotypically, zebrafish cardio-genesis has a too complex process and it also has cardiac remodeling pattern with the involvement of multiple transcription factors and cell signaling networks [47-48]. Furthermore, the zebrafish heart is more sensitive and readily engages the structural and functional defects with cardiotoxic stimuli which lead to developing the cardiac disorders via alteration of cardiac size, shape, and functions [48-49]. These all changes are able to observe with direct morphological features and simple & advanced tool in zebrafish heart. Therefore, the screening of cardiovascular drugs in a zebrafish model of CVDs is valid and acceptable methods [2]. The following section reveals the possible methods of CVDs induction in zebrafish animal.

ZEBRAFISH MODELS FOR CVDS

Defects in cardiac progenitor cells dynamics make the abnormalities of part of heart i.e., cardiac bifida, hypoplastic and hyperplastic conditions, which mainly occur via mutation of multiple cardiac-specific genes [50]. Further, the abnormalities of cardiac chamber maturation cause the hypotrabeculation and impairments the valvulogenesis [11]. And, it is altered the hemodynamic pattern. Even, it also shows the abnormal cardiac rhythmicity like arrhythmias [51]. The malfunction of the zebrafish heart occurred with both genetic and nongenetic factors. The genetic factors like cardiomyocyte functional protein gene; growth factor gene; and transcriptional factors are employed in the progression of cardiovascular defects in zebrafish [11]. These genetic factors are summarized in Table 1. Even, identical mutations of these factors are causing multiple cardiac dysfunctions [52].

Furthermore, certain non-genetic factors are also employed in the modulation of zebrafish cardiac morphogenesis via perturbing genetic networks [75]. Moreover, non-genetic factors are further categorized based on their function on the changes of hemodynamic flow and toxic effects on cardiomyocytes [25, 76]. The application of mechanical events has been producing the major changes in zebrafish cardiac blood flow and cardiac structural malformations. The mechanical events such as shear stress (frictional force between blood and walls of the blood vessels); a stretch of the blood vessels; and cardiac chamber pressure alter the homeostasis of cardiac function [77]. In zebrafish animal, the trabeculation step is highly sensitive with flow pattern and it has an additional relationship with magnitude and directionality of between blood flow; and valvulogenesis[78]. Recently, various researchers have identified the multiple pharmacological agents involved in the progression of CVDs in different stages of zebrafish embryo and adult zebrafish. The following methods are very commonly employed for the screening of novel lead molecules in zebrafish heart models. Such methods are endocrine disruptors;[21] cigarette smoke (CS; nicotine) condensate;[22] acrylamide (AA);[35-36, 79] phthalates and phosphate (P&P);[23] heavy metals;[25] inoculation infectious agent (dsRed *M. marinum*);[24] alcohol;[80] surgery (cryosection & amputation);[18, 26] and laser light radiations.[81] Various methods are identified in the progression of cardiovascular toxicity in zebrafish embryos and adult zebrafish with multiple genetic and non-genetic factors. This book chapter also covers the cell signaling, molecular mechanisms, morphological, functional, physiological, electrophysiological and histopathological based changes of zebrafish heart.

Table 1. List of genetic factor is involved in morphogenesis of zebrafish myocardium

Genetic factors	Genes	Effects on myocardium	References
Functional protein gene	MYH6	Atrial contraction	[53-54]
	ACTC	Endocardial cushion morphogenesis	[27, 55]
	TITIN	Sarcomere assembly	[56-57]
	KCNH2	Ventricular asystole, QT intreval	[58-59]
Growth factor gene	NOTCH1	Valvulogenesis, conduction tissue specification, trabeculation	[60-61]
	SMAD6	CM proliferation	[62-63]
	FLK1	Valvulogenesis	[64-65]
	SEMA3	Primary heart field size	[23, 66]
Transcriptional factors	GATA4/5/6	Modification of CM specification	[67-68]
	NKX2.5	Looping, CM proliferation, CM differentiation	[69-70]
	TBX5	Bradycardia, looping	[71-72]
	HAND2	Cardiac differentiation	[73-74]

Abbreviation:ACTC, Alpha-cardiac actin; FLK1,vascular endothelial growth factor (VEGF); CM, cardiomyocyte; GATA4/5/6,GATA, erythroid transcription factor; GATA4 transcription factor; HAND2, Helix-loop-helix transcription factor; KCNH2,potassium channel, voltage-gated EAG related subfamily H, member 2; MYH6, Alpha-myosin heavy chain; NKX2.5,Homeobox containing transcription factor 2-5; NOTCH1,Notch homolog1; SEMA3,Semaphorin 3; SMAD, human homologue of Mad and Sma proteins; SMAD6, SMAD family member 6; TBX5,T-box 5 transcription factor; and TITIN, Titin.

The administration of endocrine disruptors i.e., bisphenol-A(BPA: 0.2, 0.6, 1.7, 2.9, 5.7, 11.5, 23.0 and 45 μM); bisphenol AF (BPAF: 0.2, 0.6, 1.8, 5.2, 15.3 and 45 μM); bisphenol B (BPB); bisphenol F (BPF: 0.6, 1.7, 5.1, 15 and 44 μM) and bisphenol S (BPS: 0.2, 0.6, 1.8, 5.2, 15.3 and 45μM) produce the alteration of zebrafish specific estrogen receptor β_2 (zfER-β_2) activity in 10 dpf embryos. Further, these agents have shown decreased locomotor activity, heart rate, and hatching rate; reduced ventricular beats and blood flow [11, 21, 82]. Further, the exposure of cigarette smoke (CS, nicotine condensate) extract in 4 hpf embryo, and 3-18 months old adult male and female transgenic zebrafish enhanced green fluorescent protein (Fli1a: EGF) with rising of myocardial oxidative stress and neuronal impulse; activation of nicotinic receptors; and reduction of antioxidant defense enzymes. Moreover, 1:4 and 1:30 dilution of CS (60 snuff packs) exposure for 24 and 48 hours in embryo and one week exposure in adult enhances the mortality rate, decrease the hatching rate, reduction of ventricular mass and dimensions, lowers the heart rate, stroke volume and cardiac output [22, 83]. Further, roasted potato based toxic chemicals i.e., like acrylamide (ACR: 0.5–1.0 mM of ACR for 7 days) exposure in 1 hpf showed shortened the ventricular fraction, develop the ellipsoid structure of heart, decreased volume of blood flow, defect of cardiac looping, raised pericardial edema, developed cardiac hypertrophy and collapsed blood circulation along with reduction of heart rate without alteration of atrial and ventricular rate [35-36, 79].

In addition, phosphate and phthalate (P & P) i.e., triphenyl phosphate (TPP), dibutyl phthalate (DBP: 0.36, 1.8 and 3.6 μM) and butyl benzyl phthalate (BBP: 0.1, 0.6 and 1.2 mg/L) in 4 to 72 hpf embryos showed the rising of cardio-specific genes i.e., Nkx2.5 and T-box transcription factor 5 expression; activates the retinoic acid receptor (RAR) subtypes like RARα, RARβ and RARγ; inhibits the RA-induced luciferase activity; and induces the yolk-sac edema. Furthermore, P&P also reduces the embryo development; abnormal spinal curvature, tail deformity, uninflated swim bladder, and cardiac defects; decreased body length and heart rate; and reduced the distance between SV and BA [23, 84-85]. The exposure of heavy metals like arsenic (50, 100, 300 and 500 ppb 72 hours), cadmium

(100 μM), lead and copper (0.1 mg/ml) in 5 to 72 hpf embryos and adult zebrafish (50 to 300 ppb of arsenic for 6 months) elevates the superoxide dismutase (SOD) protein levels; raises the oxidative stress and increased genetic and/or epigenetic changes. Moreover, heavy metals are also reduced the heart rate; locomotion; defects of dorsal aortae & vascular system; and raises the mortality, heart rate and body length [25, 86-88]. The inoculation of infectious agent i.e., dsRed *M. marinum* [20 nl of 20 ng/ml of *M. tuberculi* strain injected with H37RV to macrophage colony-stimulating factor (MCSF)] in 48 hpf embryos with rising of free radicals, cytokines and autacoids which leads to defects of caudal vein, reduces the blood circulation, raising of mortality, alteration of swim bladder structure, abnormalities of swim bladder, discoloration of yolk and raised the pericardial edemas [24, 89]. Further, the alcohol (30% v/v ethanol for 24 hours) exposure of 54 to 72 hpf embryos raises the free radicals and oxidative stress on myocardial tissue. And, it reduces the heart rates, ventricular thickness, functional maturity, cardiac conducting system and increased heart volumes [80, 90].

A recent method of CVD models of zebrafish is myocardial injury via amputation of cardiac tissue, cryoinjury (CI) and laser radiation [91-93]. The surgical removal of myocardial with cold injury developed CVDs in 18 months old adult male and female zebrafish. The liquid nitrogen (-210°C at room temperature) cooled copper probe applied on the ventricle (25% area) followed by dissected scar tissue of myocardium at 1 and 4 dpi. The elevation of free radicals makes the irreversible injury leads to raises the cardiac myocyte proliferation and alters the rate of regeneration of cardiac muscles [18]. Furthermore, ventricular apex and 20% ventricular amputation in 3 months old adult zebrafish accelerates the free radicals, cytokines, autacoids generations, rising of collagen deposition, enhances the expression of periostin-b, fibronectin, and tenascin-C in epicardium tissue [26].

Table 2. Summary of zebrafish models for CVDs

Sl. No	Compounds	Animals	Dose/action	Mechanisms	Assessments	References
	Endocrine disruptors (BPA; BPAF; BPB; BPF; and BPS).	10 dpf embryos.	• 0.2, 0.6, 1.7, 2.9, 5.7, 11.5, 23.0 and 45 μM of BPA; 0.2, 0.6, 1.8, 5.2, 15.3 and 45μM of BPAF; 0.6, 1.7, 5.1, 15 and 44μM of BPB; 0.2, 0.6, 1.8, 5.2, 15.3 and 45μM of BPF; and 0.2, 0.6, 1.8, 5.2, 15.3 and 45μM of BPS.	• Altered zfER specifically zfER-β2 activity.	• Decreased locomotor activity. • Reduced heart rate and hatching rate. • Reduced ventricular beats and blood flow.	[11, 21, 82]
	CS (nicotine condensate)	4 hpf embryo. 3-18 months old adult male and female transgenic zebrafish (Fli1a: EGF).	• Exposed 1:4 and 1:30 dilution of CS (60 snuff packs) for 24 and 48 hours. • Adult exposed 1 week.	• Induced oxidative stress. • Decreased anti-oxidant defense enzymes. • Enhanced the neuronal impulse. • Activated the nicotinic receptors.	• Increased 73 percentages of 4 hpf embryos. • Decreased hatching rate. • Reduced ventricular dimensions. • Lowered heart rate, stroke volume, and cardiac output.	[22, 83]
	AA (ACR)	1 hpf of embryos.	• Exposed 0.5–1.0 mM of ACR for 7 days.	• Increased free radicals. • Reduced anti-oxidant synthesis i.e., reduced glutathione. • Interfere with gene functions.	• Shortened ventricular fraction and ellipsoid structure of the heart. Decreased volume of blood flow. Defected cardiac looping. Raised pericardial edema. • Developed cardiac hypertrophy and collapsed blood circulation. • Half reduction of heart rate; no changes of atrial and ventricular rate.	[35-36]

Table 2. (Continued)

Sl. No	Compounds	Animals	Dose/action	Mechanisms	Assessments	References
	P&P (TPP, DBP and BBP)	4 to 72 hpf embryos.	• Exposed 0.36, 1.8 and 3.6 μM of DBP. • Exposed 0.1, 0.6 and 1.2 mg/L of BBP for 72 hpf.	• Increased expression of cardiogenic genes i.e., Nkx2.5 and T-box transcription factor 5. • Activated RAR_{α}, RAR_{β}andRAR_{γ} • Inhibited RA-induced luciferase activity.	• Induced yolk-sac edema. • Decreased embryo development. • Abnormal spinal curvature, tail deformity, uninflated swim bladder, and cardiac defects. • Decreased body length and heart rate. • Reduced distance between SV and BA.	[23, 84-85]
	Heavy metals (Arsenic, cadmium, lead, and copper)	5 to 72hpfembryos. Adult zebrafish.	• Exposed 50, 100, 300 and 500 ppb of arsenic for 72 hours. • Exposed 50 to 300 ppb of arsenic for 6 months. • Exposed 100 micro M cadmium. • Exposed 1mg/ml of lead and 0.1 mg/ml of copper sulfate.	• Elevated SOD protein levels. • Increased oxidative stress. • Induced genetic and/or epigenetic changes.	• Decreased heart rate. • Decrease locomotion. • Localized defects of dorsal aortae and vascular system. • Increased mortality, heart rate, and body length.	[25, 86-88]
	Infectious agent (dsRed*M. marinum*)	48 hpf embryos.	• 20 nl of 20 ng/ml of M.tuberculosis strain injected with H37RV to MCSF.	• Enhanced free radicals. • Raised the cytokines and autacoids.	• Defects of the caudal vein. Reduced blood circulation. Increased mortality. • Alters the structure of swim bladder • Inflation of swim bladder. Discoloration of yolk. Raised pericardial edemas.	[24, 89]
	Alcohol (Ethanol)	54 to 72 hpfembryos.	• Exposed 30% v/v of ethanol solution for 24 hours.	• Maybe raised the free radicals. • Alteration of cellular enzymatic system.	• Decreased heart rates, ventricular thickness, functional maturity, and cardiac conducting system. • Increased heart volumes.	[80, 90]

Sl. No	Compounds	Animals	Dose/action	Mechanisms	Assessments	Refe-rences
	Surgery	Cold injury + Amputation: 18 months old adult male and female zebrafish.	• Liquid nitrogen cooled copper probe applied on the ventricle (25% area). • Removed scar tissue after CI on 1 and 4 dpi.	• Controlled free radical generated for irreversible injury.	• Observed the rate of cardiac myocyte proliferation. • Rate of regeneration of damaged tissue was noted. • Morphogenesis of normal heart was observed.	[18]
		Ventricular apex amputation: >3 months old zebrafish	• Removed apex part of zebrafish ventricle.	• Accelerated the free radicals, cytokines, and autacoids. • Expressed collagen and matrix metalloproteins.	• Increased collagen deposition. Enhanced expression of periostin-b,fibronectin, and tenascin-C in epicardium of 30 dpa. • Induced regeneration of heart tissues within 50 dpa.	[26]
		20% ventricular amputation:Adult zebrafish, 3-4 cm in length.	• Removed 20% of zebrafish ventricle.	• Accelerated the free radicals, cytokines, and autacoids. • Induced expression of collagen and matrix metallo proteins.	• Induced distinct P waves, QRS complexes and QT intervals within 4 dpa. • Reduced heart rate. Histology revealed apical thrombi replaced with fibrin clots and collagen fibers.	[94]
	Radiation (Synchronized laser light)	72 hpfembryos.	• Laser passed to specific region i.e., apex-ventricle, AV and BA.	• Dysfunction developed 2 to 24 hours post-injury (hpi).	• Apex: Reduced ventricle ejection fraction (EF) at 24 hpi. • Ventricle and near AV: Developed bradycardia and atrial-ventricular dysfunction. Direct AV cushion: Regurgitation of blood from the ventricle to atrium. BA: Obstructed temporary outflow tract with the cessation of ventricle contraction and blood circulation.	[81]

Abbreviation: AA, acrylic amide; ACR, acrylamide; BA, bulbus arteriosus; BBP, butyl benzyl phthalate; BPA, bisphenol-A; BPAF, bisphenol AF; BPB, bisphenol B; BPF, bisphenol F; BPS, bisphenol S; CS, cigarette smoke; DA, diterpene alkaloids; DAU, daunorubicin; DBP, dibutyl phthalate; dpa, days post-amputation; dpf, days post-fertilization; EF, ejection fraction; EGFP, enhanced green fluorescent protein; hpf, hours post-fertilization; hpi, hours post injury; MCSF, macrophage colony-stimulating factor; Nkx2.5, cardiac-specific homeobox 1; P&P, phthalatesand phosphate; RA, retinoic acid; RAR, retinoic acidreceptor; RXR, retinoid receptors; SV, sinus venosus; T-box-5, T-box transcription factor 5; TPP, triphenyl phosphate; zfER, zebrafish specific estrogen receptor; and zfER-β_2, zebrafish specific estrogen β_2 receptor.

In addition, myocardial injury also alters the electrocardiogram (ECG) waves i.e., P waves, QRS complexes and QT intervals and reduces the heart rate along with the formation of apical thrombi [94]. The application of synchronized laser light radiation in 72 hpf embryos and specific regions of adult zebrafish myocardium i.e., apex-ventricle, AV and BA showed myocardial dysfunction within 2 to 24 hours post-injury (hpi). The apex radiation causes reduction of ventricle ejection fraction (EF) at 24 hpi; ventricle and near AV injury showed bradycardia and AV dysfunction; direct injury of AV cushion produced regurgitation of blood from ventricle to atrium; and BA injury shown obstruction of temporary outflow tract with cessation of ventricle contraction and blood circulation [81]. Based on above the literature reports, the zebrafish models have been considered as a major species for the screening of novel lead molecules for CVDs. The summary of zebrafish CVDs models is listed in Table 2.

Conclusion

The various methods are inducing the CVDs in the zebrafish embryo and adult zebrafish. The external development of zebrafish heart is one of the major advantages for the analysis of congenital heart disease and changes cardiac morphogenesis. The primary mechanism of endocrine disruptor's associated cardiac morphogenesis is due to the alteration of zfER-β_2 activity. Further, the acceleration of free radicals generations, decreasing of endogenous anti-oxidant molecules like reduced glutathione are involved in ACR, heavy metal, alcohol, and radiation-induced CVDs in zebrafish. In addition to free radicals generation and immunological alterations are also involved in infectious and cigarette smoke associated CVDs. The exposure of P&P substances have elevated the expression of Nkx2.5 & T-box-5 transcription factors; activates the RAR subfamilies i.e., RARα, RARβ & RARγ; and inhibits the RA associated luciferase activity. Based on this book chapter information can make understanding the morphogenesis of zebrafish heart, advantages, and limitation of CVDs study in zebrafish, method of induction of CVDs in zebrafish and embryos, essential molecular toxic mechanisms and involvement of genetic modifications. This is the first report to summarized data for the induction of CVDs in zebrafish and the molecular target of CVD progression in zebrafish. In addition, it also covers the possible assessment parameters on zebrafish cardiac morphogenesis, functional abnormalities, changes of electrophysiological and histopathological parameters, possible modification of genetic materials and possibilities to study of cardiac regeneration properties.

FUTURE DIRECTIONS

The wide area of CVDs in zebrafish models with basic cardiac and valvulogenesis makes a clear understanding of CVDs models, mechanisms and their targets. Hence, it can lead to newer development and screening of lead molecules for CVDs drug discovery and make the successful molecule to clinical setup. The major point of zebrafish external cardio morphogenesis can lead to the discovery of medicine for congenital heart disease and overcome the rodent research associated limitation of drug discovery. So that, zebrafish models for screening of cardiotoxic agents can exist the ambit of cardiovascular research.

REFERENCES

[1] Mc Namara, K., Alzubaidi, H. and Jackson, J. K. (2019). Cardiovascular disease as a leading cause of death: how are pharmacists getting involved? *Integr Pharm Res Pract,* 8: 1.

[2] Giardoglou, P. and Beis, D. (2019). On zebrafish disease models and matters of the heart. *Biomedicines*, 7(1): 15.

[3] Savoji, H., Mohammadi, M. H., Rafatian, N., Toroghi, M. K., Wang, E. Y., Zhao, Y., Korolj, A., Ahadian, S. and Radisic, M. (2019). Cardiovascular disease models: A game changing paradigm in drug discovery and screening. *Biomaterials,* 198: 3-26.

[4] Bala, S., Pathak, R. K. and Mishra, V. (2011). Identification of EPAC (Exchange protein activated by cAMP) bioinformatically as a potential signalling biomarker in cardiovascular disease (CVD) and its molecular docking by a lead molecule. *Bioinformation,* 6(5): 176-178.

[5] Vilar, S., Sobarzo-Sanchez, E., Santana, L. and Uriarte, E. (2017). Molecular docking and drug discovery in beta-adrenergic receptors. *Curr Med Chem,* 24(39): 4340-4359.

[6] Niu, J., Straubinger, R. M. and Mager, D. E. (2019). Pharmacodynamic drug-drug interactions. *Clin Pharmacol Ther.*

[7] Uddin, M. E., Sun, X., Huang, K. M., Hu, S., Carnes, C. A., Sparreboom, A. and Fu, Q. (2019). Development and validation of a UPLC-MS/MS analytical method for dofetilide in mouse plasma and urine, and its application to pharmacokinetic study. *J Pharm Biomed Anal.*

[8] Cops, J., Haesen, S., De Moor, B., Mullens, W. and Hansen, D. (2019). Current animal models for the study of congestion in heart failure: an overview. *Heart Fail Rev,* 1-11.

[9] Leong, X. F., Ng, C. Y. and Jaarin, K. (2015). Animal models in cardiovascular research: Hypertension and atherosclerosis. *Biomed Res Int,* 2015: 528757.

[10] Zhong, Y., Huang, W., Du, J., Wang, Z., He, J. and Luo, L. (2019). Improved Tol2-mediated enhancer trap identifies weakly expressed genes during liver and β cell development and regeneration in zebrafish. *J Biol Chem.* 294(3): 932-940.

[11] Brown, D., Samsa, L., Qian, L. and Liu, J. (2016). Advances in the study of heart development and disease using zebrafish. *J Cardiovasc Dev Dis,* 3(2): 13.

[12] Genge, C. E., Lin, E., Lee, L., Sheng, X., Rayani, K., Gunawan, M., Stevens, C. M., Li, A. Y., Talab, S. S., Claydon, T. W., Hove-Madsen, L. and Tibbits, G. F. (2016). The zebrafish heart as a model of mammalian cardiac function. *Rev Physiol Biochem Pharmacol*, 171: 99-136.

[13] Pestel, J., Ramadass, R., Gauvrit, S., Helker, C., Herzog, W. and Stainier, D. Y. (2016). Real-time 3D visualization of cellular

rearrangements during cardiac valve formation. *Development*, 143(12): 2217-2227.

[14] Vornanen, M. and Hassinen, M. (2016). Zebrafish heart as a model for human cardiac electrophysiology. *Channels*, 10(2): 101-110.

[15] Rissone, A. and Burgess, S. M. (2018). Rare genetic blood disease modeling in zebrafish. *Front Genet,* 9: 348.

[16] Geary, B., Magee, K., Cash, P., Husi, H., Young, I. S., Whitfield, P. D. and Doherty, M. K. (2019). Acute stress alters the rates of degradation of cardiac muscle proteins. *J Proteomic,* 191: 124-130.

[17] Hirose, K., Payumo, A. Y., Cutie, S., Hoang, A., Zhang, H., Guyot, R., Lunn, D., Bigley, R. B., Yu, H. and Wang, J. (2019). Evidence for hormonal control of heart regenerative capacity during endothermy acquisition. *Science,* EAAR 2038.

[18] Gonzalez-Rosa, J. M. and Mercader, N. (2012). Cryoinjury as a myocardial infarction model for the study of cardiac regeneration in the zebrafish. *Nat Protoc,* 7(4): 782-788.

[19] Ellison, D. H. (2019).Mechanistic insights into loop diuretic responsiveness in heart failure. *Am Soc Nephrol.*

[20] Kunisaki, S. M. (2012). Congenital anomalies: treatment options based on amniotic fluid-derived stem cells. *Organogenesis,* 8(3): 89-95.

[21] Catron, T. R., Keely, S. P., Brinkman, N. E., Zurlinden, T. J., Wood, C. E., Wright, J. R., Phelps, D., Wheaton, E., Kvasnicka, A., Gaballah, S., Lamendella, R. and Tal, T. (2019). Host developmental toxicity of BPA and BPA alternatives is inversely related to microbiota disruption in zebrafish. *Toxicol Sci,* 167(2): 468-483.

[22] Folkesson, M., Sadowska, N., Vikingsson, S., Karlsson, M., Carlhall, C. J., Lanne, T., Wagsater, D. and Jensen, L. (2016). Differences in cardiovascular toxicities associated with cigarette smoking and snuff use revealed using novel zebrafish models. *Biol Open*, 5(7): 970-978.

[23] Sun, G. and Liu, K. (2017). Developmental toxicity and cardiac effects of butyl benzyl phthalate in zebrafish embryos. *Aquat Toxicol,* 192: 165-170.

[24] Vibe, C. B., Fenaroli, F., Pires, D., Wilson, S. R., Bogoeva, V., Kalluru, R., Speth, M., Anes, E., Griffiths, G. and Hildahl, J. (2016). Thioridazine in PLGA nanoparticles reduces toxicity and improves rifampicin therapy against mycobacterial infection in zebrafish. *Nanotoxicology*, 10(6): 680-688.

[25] Zakaria, Z. Z., Benslimane, F. M., Nasrallah, G. K., Shurbaji, S., Younes, N. N., Mraiche, F., Da'as, S. I. and Yalcin, H. C. (2018). Using zebrafish for investigating the molecular mechanisms of drug-induced cardiotoxicity. *Bio Med Res Int,* 2018.

[26] Ito, K., Morioka, M., Kimura, S., Tasaki, M., Inohaya, K. and Kudo, A. (2014). Differential reparative phenotypes between zebrafish and medaka after cardiac injury. *Dev Dyn,* 243(9): 1106-1115.

[27] Grant, M. G., Patterson, V. L., Grimes, D. T. and Burdine, R. D. (2017). Modeling syndromic congenital heart defects in zebrafish. *Curr Top Dev Biol*, 124: 1-40.

[28] Yan, Z., Huang, X., Xie, Y., Song, M., Zhu, K. and Ding, S. (2019). Macrolides induce severe cardiotoxicity and developmental toxicity in zebrafish embryos. *Sci Total Environ,* 649: 1414-1421.

[29] Hill, J. T., Demarest, B., Gorsi, B., Smith, M. and Yost, H. J. (2017). Heart morphogenesis gene regulatory networks revealed by temporal expression analysis. *Development,* 144(19): 3487-3498.

[30] Sánchez-Iranzo, H., Galardi-Castilla, M., Minguillón, C., Sanz-Morejón, A., González-Rosa, J. M., Felker, A., Ernst, A., Guzmán-Martínez, G., Mosimann, C. and Mercader, N. (2018). Tbx5a lineage tracing shows cardiomyocyte plasticity during zebrafish heart regeneration. *Nat Commun* 9(1): 428.

[31] Tekeli, I., Garcia-Puig, A., Notari, M., Garcia-Pastor, C., Aujard, I., Jullien, L. and Raya, A. (2017). Fate predetermination of cardiac myocytes during zebrafish heart regeneration. *Open Biol*, 7(6).

[32] Mishra, S., Joshi, S., Ward, J. E., Buys, E. P., Mishra, D., Mishra, D., Morgado, I., Fisch, S., Lavatelli, F. and Merlini, G. (2019). Zebrafish model of amyloid light chain cardiotoxicity: regeneration vs degeneration. *Am J Physiol Heart Circ Physiol.*

[33] Qian, L., Qi, S., Cao, F., Zhang, J., Li, C., Song, M. and Wang, C. (2019). Effects of penthiopyrad on the development and behaviour of zebrafish in early-life stages. *Chemosphere,* 214: 184-194.

[34] Katano, W., Moriyama, Y., Takeuchi, J. K. and Koshiba-Takeuchi, K. (2019). Cardiac septation in heart development and evolution. *Dev Growth Differ,* 61(1): 114-123.

[35] Huang, M., Jiao, J., Wang, J., Xia, Z. and Zhang, Y. (2018b). Exposure to acrylamide induces cardiac developmental toxicity in zebrafish during cardiogenesis. *Environ Pollut*, 234: 656-666.

[36] Huang, M., Zhu, F., Jiao, J., Wang, J. and Zhang, Y. (2019). Exposure to acrylamide disrupts cardiomyocyte interactions during ventricular morphogenesis in zebrafish embryos. *Sci Total Environ,* 656: 1337-1345.

[37] Han, Y., Chen, A., Umansky, K.-B., Oonk, K. A., Choi, W.-Y., Dickson, A. L., Ou, J., Cigliola, V., Yifa, O. and Cao, J. (2019). Vitamin D stimulates cardiomyocyte proliferation and controls organ size and regeneration in zebrafish. *Dev Cell.*

[38] Jiménez-Amilburu, V. and Stainier, D. Y. (2019). The transmembrane protein Crb2a regulates cardiomyocyte apicobasal polarity and adhesion in zebrafish. *Dev,* 171207.

[39] Pawlak, M., Kedzierska, K. Z., Migdal, M., Nahia, K. A., Ramilowski, J. A., Bugajski, L., Hashimoto, K., Marconi, A., Piwocka, K. and Carninci, P. (2019). Dynamics of cardiomyocyte transcriptome and chromatin landscape demarcates key events of heart development. *Genome Res,* 29(3): 506-519.

[40] Li, L., Ning, G., Yang, S., Yan, Y., Cao, Y. and Wang, Q. (2019b). BMP signaling is required for nkx2. 3-positive pharyngeal pouch progenitor specification in zebrafish. *PLoS Genet,* 15(2): e1007996.

[41] Zhao, L., Ben-Yair, R., Burns, C. E. and Burns, C. G. (2019). Endocardial notch signaling promotes cardiomyocyte proliferation in the regenerating zebrafish heart through Wnt pathway antagonism. *Cell Rep,* 26(3): 546-554. e545.

[42] Wu, Y., Zhang, Y., Chen, M., Yang, Q., Zhuang, S., Lv, L., Zuo, Z. and Wang, C. (2019). Exposure to low-level metalaxyl impacts the

cardiac development and function of zebrafish embryos. *J Environ Sci.*

[43] Battista, N. A., Douglas, D. R., Lane, A. N., Samsa, L. A., Liu, J. and Miller, L. A. (2019). Vortex dynamics in trabeculated embryonic ventricles. *J Cardiovasc Dev Dis,* 6(1): 6.

[44] Colliva, A., Braga, L., Giacca, M. and Zacchigna, S. (2019). Endothelial-cardiomyocyte cross-talk in heart development and disease. *J Physiol.*

[45] Faucherre, A., ou Maati, H. M., Nasr, N., Pinard, A., Theron, A., Odelin, G., Desvignes, J. P., Salgado, D., Beroud, G. C. and Avierinos, J. F. (2019). Piezo1 is required for outflow tract and aortic valve development. *BioRxiv,* 528588.

[46] Li, J., Yue, Y. and Zhao, Q. (2016a). Retinoic acid signaling is essential for valvulogenesis by affecting endocardial cushions formation in zebrafish embryos. *Zebrafish*, 13(1): 9-18.

[47] Nakajima, Y. (2019). Retinoic acid signaling in heart development. *Genesis,* e23300.

[48] van Opbergen, C. J., van der Voorn, S. M., Vos, M. A., de Boer, T. P. and van Veen, T. A. (2018). Cardiac Ca 2+ signalling in zebrafish: Translation of findings to man. *Prog Biophys Mol Biol.*

[49] Song, G., Han, M., Li, Z., Gan, X., Chen, X., Yang, J., Dong, S., Yan, M., Wan, J. and Wang, Y. (2018). Deletion of Pr72 causes cardiac developmental defects in Zebrafish. *PLoS One*, 13(11): e0206883.

[50] Chen, B. (2018).GATA transcription factors and cardiovascular disease. In *Heart Genomics,* 127-151: Springer Nature Singapore Pte Ltd., Singapore. eBook ISBN: 978-981-13-1429-2.

[51] Bournele, D. and Beis, D. (2016). Zebrafish models of cardiovascular disease. *Heart Fail Rev,* 21(6): 803-813.

[52] Da'as, S. I., Thanassoulas, A., Calver, B. L., Beck, K., Salem, R., Saleh, A., Kontogianni, I., Al-Maraghi, A., Nasrallah, G. K. and Safieh-Garabedian, B. (2019). Arrhythmogenic calmodulin E105A mutation alters cardiac RyR2 regulation leading to cardiac dysfunction in zebrafish. *Ann N Y Acad Sci.*

[53] Berdougo, E., Coleman, H., Lee, D. H., Stainier, D. Y. and Yelon, D. (2003). Mutation of weak atrium/atrial myosin heavy chain disrupts atrial function and influences ventricular morphogenesis in zebrafish. *Development*, 130(24): 6121-6129.

[54] Jin, D., Ni, T. T., Hou, J., Rellinger, E. and Zhong, T. P. (2009). Promoter analysis of ventricular myosin heavy chain (vmhc) in zebrafish embryos. *Dev Dyn*, 238(7): 1760-1767.

[55] Glenn, N. O., McKane, M., Kohli, V., Wen, K. K., Rubenstein, P. A., Bartman, T. and Sumanas, S. (2012). The W-loop of alpha-cardiac actin is critical for heart function and endocardial cushion morphogenesis in zebrafish. *Mol Cell Biol*, 32(17): 3527-3540.

[56] Seeley, M., Huang, W., Chen, Z., Wolff, W. O., Lin, X. and Xu, X. (2007). Depletion of zebrafish titin reduces cardiac contractility by disrupting the assembly of Z-discs and A-bands. *Circ Res*, 100(2): 238-245.

[57] Zou, J., Tran, D., Baalbaki, M., Tang, L. F., Poon, A., Pelonero, A., Titus, E. W., Yuan, C., Shi, C., Patchava, S., Halper, E., Garg, J., Movsesyan, I., Yin, C., Wu, R., Wilsbacher, L. D., Liu, J., Hager, R. L., Coughlin, S. R., Jinek, M., Pullinger, C. R., Kane, J. P., Hart, D. O., Kwok, P. Y. and Deo, R. C. (2015). An internal promoter underlies the difference in disease severity between N- and C-terminal truncation mutations of Titin in zebrafish. *Elife*, 4: e09406.

[58] Arnaout, R., Ferrer, T., Huisken, J., Spitzer, K., Stainier, D. Y., Tristani-Firouzi, M. and Chi, N. C. (2007). Zebrafish model for human long QT syndrome. *Proc Natl Acad Sci USA*, 104(27): 11316-11321.

[59] Tanaka, Y., Hayashi, K., Fujino, N., Konno, T., Tada, H., Nakanishi, C., Hodatsu, A., Tsuda, T., Nagata, Y., Teramoto, R., Yoshida, S., Nomura, A., Kawashiri, M. A. and Yamagishi, M. (2019). Functional analysis of KCNH2 gene mutations of type 2 long QT syndrome in larval zebrafish using microscopy and electrocardiography. *Heart Vessels,* 34(1): 159-166.

[60] Munch, J., Grivas, D., Gonzalez-Rajal, A., Torregrosa-Carrion, R. and de la Pompa, J. L. (2017). Notch signalling restricts inflammation and

serpine1 expression in the dynamic endocardium of the regenerating zebrafish heart. *Development,* 144(8): 1425-1440.

[61] Wang, F., Yang, Q., Wu, F., Zhang, Y., Sun, S., Wang, X., Gui, Y. and Li, Q. (2019). Identification of a 42-bp heart-specific enhancer of the notch1b gene in zebrafish embryos. *Dev Dyn.*

[62] Li, A. H., Hanchard, N. A., Azamian, M., D'Alessandro, L. C., Coban-Akdemir, Z., Lopez, K. N., Hall, N. J., Dickerson, H., Nicosia, A. and Fernbach, S. (2019a). Genetic architecture of laterality defects revealed by whole exome sequencing. *Eur J Hum Genet,* 1.

[63] Wylie, L. A., Mouillesseaux, K. P., Chong, D. C. and Bautch, V. L. (2018). Developmental SMAD6 loss leads to blood vessel hemorrhage and disrupted endothelial cell junctions. *Dev Biol,* 442(2): 199-209.

[64] Li, M., Liu, X. and Feng, X. (2019c). Cardiovascular toxicity and anxiety-like behavior induced by deltamethrin in zebrafish (Danio rerio) larvae. *Chemosphere*, 219: 155-164.

[65] Shi, X., Chen, R., Zhang, Y., Yun, J., Brand-Arzamendi, K., Liu, X. and Wen, X.-Y. (2018). Zebrafish heart failure models: opportunities and challenges. *Amino acids*, 50(7): 787-798.

[66] Minchin, J. E., Scahill, C. M., Staudt, N., Busch-Nentwich, E. M. and Rawls, J. F. (2018). Deep phenotyping in zebrafish reveals genetic and diet-induced adiposity changes that may inform disease risk. *J Lipid Res,* 59(8): 1536-1545.

[67] Holtzinger, A. and Evans, T. (2007). Gata5 and Gata6 are functionally redundant in zebrafish for specification of cardiomyocytes. *Dev Biol,* 312(2): 613-622.

[68] Jia, W., Liang, D., Li, N., Liu, M., Dong, Z., Li, J., Dong, X., Yue, Y., Hu, P. and Yao, J. (2019). Zebrafish microRNA miR-210-5p inhibits primitive myelopoiesis by silencing foxj1b and slc3a2a mRNAs downstream of gata4/5/6 transcription factor genes. *J Biol Chem,* 294(8): 2732-2743.

[69] Colombo, S., de Sena-Tomas, C., George, V., Werdich, A. A., Kapur, S., MacRae, C. A. and Targoff, K. L. (2018). Nkx genes establish

second heart field cardiomyocyte progenitors at the arterial pole and pattern the venous pole through Isl1 repression. *Development*, 145(3).

[70] Yue, Y., Jiang, M., He, L., Zhang, Z., Zhang, Q., Gu, C., Liu, M., Li, N. and Zhao, Q. (2018). The transcription factor Foxc1a in zebrafish directly regulates expression of nkx2.5, encoding a transcriptional regulator of cardiac progenitor cells. *J Biol Chem,* 293(2): 638-650.

[71] Boyle Anderson, E. A. T. and Ho, R. K. (2018). A transcriptomics analysis of the Tbx5 paralogues in zebrafish. *PLoS One*, 13(12): e0208766.

[72] Ghosh, T. K., Aparicio-Sanchez, J. J., Buxton, S., Ketley, A., Mohamed, T., Rutland, C. S., Loughna, S. and Brook, J. D. (2018). Acetylation of TBX5 by KAT2B and KAT2A regulates heart and limb development. *J Mol Cell Cardiol,* 114: 185-198.

[73] Garavito-Aguilar, Z. V., Riley, H. E. and Yelon, D. (2010). Hand2 ensures an appropriate environment for cardiac fusion by limiting Fibronectin function. *Development,* 137(19): 3215-3220.

[74] Schindler, Y. L., Garske, K. M., Wang, J., Firulli, B. A., Firulli, A. B., Poss, K. D. and Yelon, D. (2014). Hand2 elevates cardiomyocyte production during zebrafish heart development and regeneration. *Development,* 141(16): 3112-3122.

[75] Sarmah, S. and Marrs, J. A. (2016). Zebrafish as a vertebrate model system to evaluate effects of environmental toxicants on cardiac development and function. *Int J Mol Sci*, 17(12).

[76] Hoog, T. G., Fredrickson, S. J., Hsu, C.-W., Senger, S. M., Dickinson, M. E. and Udan, R. S. (2018). The effects of reduced hemodynamic loading on morphogenesis of the mouse embryonic heart. *Dev Biol,* 442(1): 127-137.

[77] Boselli, F., Freund, J. B. and Vermot, J. (2015). Blood flow mechanics in cardiovascular development. *Cell Mol Life Sci,* 72(13): 2545-2559.

[78] Steed, E., Boselli, F. and Vermot, J. (2016). Hemodynamics driven cardiac valve morphogenesis. *Biochim Biophys Acta Mol Cell Res*, 1863(7): 1760-1766.

[79] Huang, M., Jiao, J., Wang, J., Xia, Z. and Zhang, Y. (2018a). Characterization of acrylamide-induced oxidative stress and

cardiovascular toxicity in zebrafish embryos. *J Hazard Mater*, 347: 451-460.

[80] Li, X., Gao, A., Wang, Y., Chen, M., Peng, J., Yan, H., Zhao, X., Feng, X. and Chen, D. (2016b). Alcohol exposure leads to unrecoverable cardiovascular defects along with edema and motor function changes in developing zebrafish larvae. *Biol Open*, 5(8): 1128-1133.

[81] Matrone, G., Maqsood, S., Taylor, J., Mullins, J. J., Tucker, C. S. and Denvir, M. A. (2014). Targeted laser ablation of the zebrafish larval heart induces models of heart block, valvular regurgitation, and outflow tract obstruction. *Zebrafish,* 11(6): 536-541.

[82] Mu, X., Huang, Y., Li, X., Lei, Y., Teng, M., Wang, C. and Li, Y. (2018). Developmental effects and estrogenicity of bisphenol A alternatives in a zebrafish embryo model. *Environ Sci Technol,* 52(5): 3222-3231.

[83] Ellis, L. D., Soo, E. C., Achenbach, J. C., Morash, M. G. and Soanes, K. H. (2014). Use of the zebrafish larvae as a model to study cigarette smoke condensate toxicity. *PLoS One,* 9(12): e115305.

[84] Antkiewicz, D. S., Burns, C. G., Carney, S. A., Peterson, R. E. and Heideman, W. (2005). Heart malformation is an early response to TCDD in embryonic zebrafish. *Toxicol Sci,* 84(2): 368-377.

[85] Isales, G. M., Hipszer, R. A., Raftery, T. D., Chen, A., Stapleton, H. M. and Volz, D. C. (2015). Triphenyl phosphate-induced developmental toxicity in zebrafish: potential role of the retinoic acid receptor. *Aquat Toxicol*, 161: 221-230.

[86] Berghmans, S., Butler, P., Goldsmith, P., Waldron, G., Gardner, I., Golder, Z., Richards, F. M., Kimber, G., Roach, A., Alderton, W. and Fleming, A. (2008). Zebrafish based assays for the assessment of cardiac, visual and gut function potential safety screens for early drug discovery. *J Pharmacol Toxicol Methods,* 58(1): 59-68.

[87] Hallauer, J., Geng, X., Yang, H. C., Shen, J., Tsai, K. J. and Liu, Z. (2016). The effect of chronic arsenic exposure in zebrafish. *Zebrafish,* 13(5): 405-412.

[88] Li, Y., Yang, X., Chen, Z., Zhang, B., Pan, J., Li, X., Yang, F. and Sun, D. (2015). Comparative toxicity of lead (Pb(2+)), copper (Cu(2+)), and mixtures of lead and copper to zebrafish embryos on a microfluidic chip. *Biomicrofluidics,* 9(2): 024105.

[89] Takaki, K., Davis, J. M., Winglee, K. and Ramakrishnan, L. (2013). Evaluation of the pathogenesis and treatment of Mycobacterium marinum infection in zebrafish. *Nat Protoc,* 8(6): 1114-1124.

[90] Dlugos, C. A. and Rabin, R. A. (2010). Structural and functional effects of developmental exposure to ethanol on the zebrafish heart. *Alcohol Clin Exp Res,* 34(6): 1013-1021.

[91] Liu, X. X., Zhang, Y. T. and Zhang, B. (2013). A surgery protocol to construct zebrafish heart damage and regeneration model. *Yi Chuan,* 35(4): 529-532.

[92] Xu, X., Meiler, S. E., Zhong, T. P., Mohideen, M., Crossley, D. A., Burggren, W. W. and Fishman, M. C. (2002). Cardiomyopathy in zebrafish due to mutation in an alternatively spliced exon of titin. *Nat Genet,* 30(2): 205-209.

[93] Zhang, X., Beebe, T., Jen, N., Lee, C. A., Tai, Y. and Hsiai, T. K. (2015). Flexible and waterproof micro-sensors to uncover zebrafish circadian rhythms: The next generation of cardiac monitoring for drug screening. *Biosens Bioelectron* 71: 150-157.

[94] Sun, P., Zhang, Y., Yu, F., Parks, E., Lyman, A., Wu, Q., Ai, L., Hu, C. H., Zhou, Q., Shung, K., Lien, C. L. and Hsiai, T. K. (2009). Micro-electrocardiograms to study post-ventricular amputation of zebrafish heart. *Ann Biomed Eng* 37(5): 890-901.

Contents of Earlier Volumes

Horizons in World Cardiovascular Research. Volume 16

Horizons in World Cardiovascular Research. Volume 15

Horizons in World Cardiovascular Research. Volume 14

Horizons in World Cardiovascular Research. Volume 13

Horizons in World Cardiovascular Research. Volume 12

INDEX

B

C

D

E

F

G

H

I

K

L

M

N

O

P

Q

R

S

T

U

V

W

Y

Z